Handbook of
Drug Interaction
and the
Mechanism of Interaction

Handbook of
Drug Interaction
and the
Mechanism of Interaction

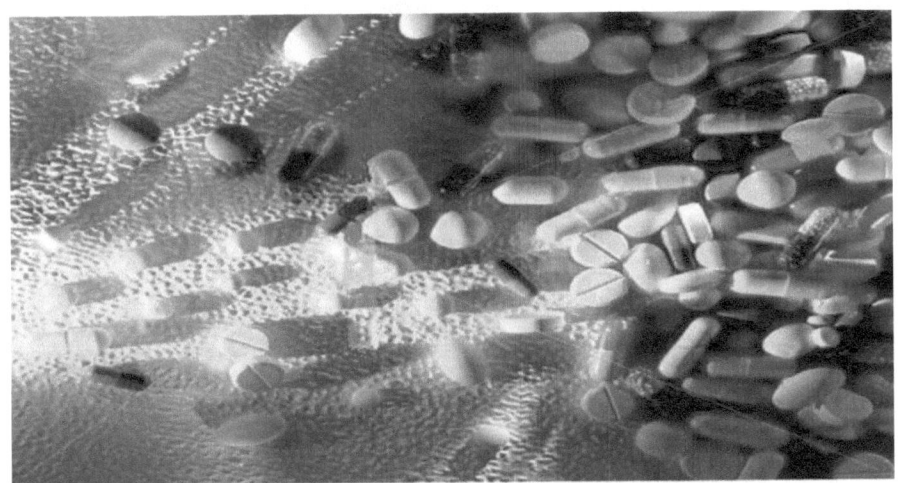

FIRST EDITION

EDITED BY

Qutaiba A. Ibrahim

MSc. Clin. Pharm. Drug Information Center (DIC), Ibn-Sena General Hospital,
Directorate of Nineveh Health, Mosul Iraq

This book was printed in the United States of America.

To order additional copies of this book, contact:
Xlibris Corporation
0-800-644-6988
www.xlibrispublishing.co.uk
Orders@xlibrispublishing.co.uk
302336

DRUG INTERACTION

Is a situation in which a substance affects the activity of a drug, i.e. the effects are increased or decreased, or they produce a new effect that neither produces on its own. Typically, interaction between drugs come to mind (drug-drug interaction). However, interactions may also exist between drugs & foods (drug-food interactions), as well as drugs & herbs (drug-herb interactions). These may occur out of accidental misuse or due to lack of knowledge about the active ingredients involved in the relevant substances.

CLINICAL IMPORTANCE OF DRUG INTERACTIONS

Clinically important adverse drug interactions become likely with the following:

- Drugs that have a steep dose-response curve and a small therapeutic index, so that relatively small quantitative changes at the target site, e.g. receptor or enzyme, will lead to substantial changes in effect, as with digoxin or lithium
- Drugs that are known enzyme inducers or inhibitors.
- Drugs that are exhibit saturable metabolism (zero-order kinetics), when small interference with kinetics may lead to large alteration of plasma concentration, e.g. phenytoin, theophylline
- Drugs that are used long-term, where precise plasma concentrations are required, e.g. oral contraceptives, antiepilepsy drugs, cardiac antiarrhythmia drugs, lithium

- When drugs that may interact are used to treat the same disease, for this increases their chance of being given concurrently, e.g. theophylline and salbutamol given for asthma may cause cardiac arrhythmia
- In severely ill patients, for they may be receiving several drugs; signs of iatrogenic disease may be difficult to distinguish from those of existing disease and the patients' condition may be such that they cannot tolerate further adversity
- In patients with significantly impaired liver or kidney function, for these are the principal organs that terminate drug action
- In the elderly, for they tend to have multiple pathology, may receive several drugs concurrently, and are specially susceptible to adverse drug effects.

What Can I Do to Help Prevent Drug Interactions?

- Before starting any new prescription drug or over-the-counter drug, talk to your primary healthcare provider or pharmacist. Make sure that they are aware of any vitamins or supplements that you take.
- Make sure to read the patient information handout given to you at the pharmacy. If you are not given an information sheet, ask your pharmacist for one.
- Check the labels of your medications for any warnings and look for the "Drug Interaction Precaution". Read these warnings carefully.
- Make a list of all your prescription medications and over-the-counter products, including drugs, vitamins, and supplements. Review this list with all healthcare providers and your pharmacist.
- If possible, use one pharmacy for all your prescription medications and over-the-counter products. This way your pharmacist has a record of all your prescription drugs and can advise you about drug interactions and side effects.

Types of Drug Interactions

Some knowledge of the pharmacological basis of how one drug may change the action of another is useful in obtaining those interactions that are wanted, as well as in recognizing and preventing those that are not.

Drug interactions are of two principal kinds:

1. Pharmacodynamic interaction:

Both drugs act on the target site of clinical effect, exerting synergism or antagonism. The drugs may act on the same or different receptors or processes, mediating similar biological consequences.

2. Pharmacokinetic interaction:

The drugs interact remotely from the target site to alter plasma (and other tissue) concentrations so that the amount of the drug at the target site of clinical effect is altered.

Antagonism occurs when the action of one drug opposes the action of another. The two drugs simply have opposite pharmacodynamic effects.

physiological or functional antagonism; or they compete reversibly for the same drug receptor.

Synergism is of two sorts:

a. Summation or addition occurs when the effects of two drugs having the same action are additive, i.e. $2 + 2 = 4$
b. Potentiation (to make more powerful) occurs when one drug increases the action of another, i.e. $2 + 2 = 5$. Sometimes the two drugs both have the action concerned (trimethoprim plus sulphonamide) and sometimes one drug lacks the action concerned (benserazide plus levodopa), i.e. $0 + 2 = 5$.

Identifying Potential Drug Interaction

Drugs can interact at any stage from when they are mixed with other drugs in a pharmaceutical formulation or by a clinician, e.g. in an i.v. infusion or syringe, to their final excretion either unchanged or as metabolites. When a drug is added to an existing regimen, a doctor can evaluate the possibility of an interaction by logically thinking through the usual sequence of processes to which a drug is subject interactions may occur:

- Outside the body
- At the site of absorption
- During distribution
- On receptors or body systems (pharmacodynamic interactions)
- During metabolism
- During excretion.

INTERACTIONS OUTSIDE THE BODY

Intravenous fluids offer special scope for interactions (incompatibilities) when drugs are added to the reservoir or syringe, for a number of reasons. Drugs commonly are weak organic acids or bases. They are often insoluble and to make them soluble it is necessary to prepare salts. Plainly, the mixing of solutions of salts can result in instability which may or may not be evident from visible change in the solution, i.e. precipitation. Furthermore, the solutions have little buffering capacity and pH readily changes with added drugs. Dilution of a drug in the reservoir fluid may also lead to loss of stability.

A serious loss of potency can result from incompatibility between an infusion fluid and a drug that is added to it. Issues of compatibility are complex but specific sources of information are available in manufacturers' package inserts, formularies or from the hospital pharmacy (where the addition ought to be made). The general rule must be to consult these sources before ever adding a drug to an infusion fluid or mixing in a syringe. Mixing drugs formulated for injection in a syringe may cause interaction.

INTERACTIONS AT SITE OF ABSORPTION

In the complex environment of the gut there are opportunities for drugs to interfere with each other both directly and indirectly via alteration of gut physiology. Usually the result is to impair absorption.

- Direct chemical interaction in the gut

Is a significant cause of reduced absorption. Antacids that contain aluminium and magnesium form insoluble complexes with tetracyclines, iron and prednisolone. Milk contains sufficient calcium to warrant its avoidance as a major article of diet when tetracyclines are taken.

Interactions of this type depend on both drugs being in the stomach at the same time, and can be prevented if the doses are separated by at least 2 hours.

Gut motility may be altered by drugs. Slowing of gastric emptying, e.g. opioid analgesics, tricyclic antidepressants (antimuscarinic effect), may delay and reduce the absorption of other drugs. Purgatives reduce the time spent in the small intestine and give less opportunity for the absorption of poorly soluble substances such as adrenal steroids and digoxin.

Alterations in gut flora by antimicrobials may potentiate oral anticoagulant by reducing bacterial synthesis of vitamin K (usually only after antimicrobials are given orally in high dose, e.g. to treat Helicobacter pylori).

Interactions other than in the gut are exemplified by the use of hyaluronidase to promote dissipation of a s.c. injection, and by the addition of vasoconstrictors, e.g. adrenaline, felypressin, to localanaesthetics to delay absorption and usefully prolong local anaesthesia.

INTERACTIONS DURING DISTRIBUTION

- Displacement from plasma protein binding sites

may contribute to adverse reaction. A drug that is extensively protein bound can be displaced from its binding site by a competing drug, so raising the free (and pharmacologically active) concentration of the first drug. Unbound drug, however, is available for distribution away from the plasma and for metabolism and excretion. Commonly, the result is that the free concentration of the displaced drug quickly returns close to its original value and any extra effect is transient.

For a displacement interaction to become clinically important, a second mechanism usually operates: sodium valproate can cause phenytoin toxicity because it both displaces phenytoin from its binding site on plasma albumin and inhibits its metabolism. Similarly aspirin and probenecid (and possibly other nonsteroidal anti-inflammatory drugs) displace the folic acid antagonist methotrexate from its protein-binding site and reduce its rate of active secretion by the renal tubules; the result is serious methotrexate toxicity.

Bilirubin is displaced from its binding protein by sulphonamides, vitamin K, X-ray contrast media or indomethacin; in the neonate this may cause a significant risk of kernicterus, for its capacity to metabolise bilirubin is immature.

Displacement from tissue binding may cause unwanted effects. When quinidine is given to patients who are receiving digoxin, the plasma concentration of free digoxin may double because quinidine displaces digoxin from binding sites in tissue (as well as plasma proteins). As with interaction due to displacement from plasma proteins, however, an additional mechanism contributes to the overall effect, for quinidine also impairs renal excretion of digoxin.

INTERACTIONS DIRECTLY ON RECEPTORS OR ON BODY SYSTEMS

This category of pharmacodynamic interactions comprises specific interactions between drugs on the same receptor, and includes less precise interactions involving the same body organ or system; whatever the precise location, the result is altered drug action.

- Action on receptors provides numerous examples.

Beneficial interactions are sought in overdose, as with the use of naloxone for morphine overdose (opioid receptor), of atropine for anticholinesterase, i.e. insecticide poisoning (acetylcholine receptor), of isoproterelol (isoprenaline) for overdose with a b-adrenoceptor blocker (b-adrenoceptor), of phentolamine for the monoamine oxidase inhibitorsympathomimetic interaction (—adrenoceptor).

Unwanted interactions include the loss of the antihypertensive effect of b-blockers when common cold remedies containing ephedrine, phenylpropanolamine or phenylephrine are taken, usually unknown to the doctor; their—adrenoceptor agonist action is unrestrained in the b-blocked patient.

- Actions on body systems provide scope for a variety of interactions.

The following list shows something of the range of possibilities; others may be found under accounts of individual drugs:

β-adrenoceptor blockers lose some antihypertensive efficacy when nonsteroidal anti-inflammatory drugs (NSAIDs), especially indomethacin, are coadministered; the effect involves inhibition of production of vasodilator prostaglandins by the kidney leading to sodium retention.

Diuretics, especially of the loop variety, lose efficacy if administered with NSAIDs; the mechanism may involve inhibition of prostaglandin synthesis, as above.

Potassium supplements, given with potassium retaining diuretics, e.g. amiloride, spironolactone, or with ACE-inhibitors may cause dangerous hyperkalaemia.

INTERACTIONS DURING METABOLISM

- Enzyme induction by drugs and other substances accelerates metabolism and is a cause of therapeutic failure. The following are examples:

Oral contraceptive steroids are metabolised more rapidly when an enzyme inducer, e.g. phenytoin, is added, and unplanned pregnancy has occurred (doctors have been successfully sued for negligence). In this circumstance an oral contraceptive of high oestrogen content may be substituted (or an alternative contraceptive method); if breakthrough bleeding occurs, the oestrogen content is not high enough. The metabolism of progestogens is also increased by enzyme induction.

- Enzyme inhibition by drugs potentiates other drugs that are inactivated by metabolism, causing adverse reactions.

Examples appear below, and it will be noted that inhibitors of isoenzymes of microsomal cytochrome P450 figure prominently. The drugs with which they interact are also given but the list is not complete, and there should be a general awareness of the possibility of metabolic inhibition when the following drugs are used.

Cimetidine is an inhibitor of several cytochrome P450 isoenzymes and so potentiates a large number of drugs ordinarily metabolized by that system, notably, theophylline, warfarin, phenytoin and propranolol. Depending on the interacting drug, up to 50% inhibition of metabolism may occur when cimetidine 2000 mg/d is taken.

Erythromycin inhibits a cytochrome P450 isoenzyme and impairs the metabolism of theophylline, warfarin, carbamazepine and methylprednisolone. The mean reduction in drug clearance is 20-25%.

INTERACTIONS DURING EXCRETION

Clinically important interactions, both beneficial and potentially harmful, occur in the kidney.

- Interference with passive diffusion

Reabsorption of a drug by the renal tubule can be reduced, and its excretion increased, by altering urine pH .

- Interference with active transport.

Organic acids are passed from the blood into the urine by active transport across the renal tubular epithelium.

Penicillin is mostly excreted in this way. Probenecid, an organic acid that competes successfully with penicillin for this transport system, may be used to prolong the action of penicillin when repeated administration is impracticable, e.g. in sexually transmitted diseases, where compliance is notoriously poor. Interference with renal excretion of methotrexate by aspirin, of zidovudine by probenecid and of digoxin by quinidine, contribute to the potentially harmful interactions with these combinations

ANTIMICROBIAL AGENTS

ANTIBACTERIAL

Aminoglycosides: Amikacin, Gentamicin, Kanamycin, Neomycin, Streptomycin, Tobramycin

DRUG	DRUG INTERACTION	EFFECT	MECHANISM OF INTERACTION
Aminoglycoside	AbobotulinumtoxinA	Increase neuromuscular—blocking effect of AbobotulinumtoxinA	Synergistic neuromuscular—blocking activity
	Amphotericin B	Increased risk of nephrotoxicity	Synergistic nephrotoxicity
	BCG	Decrease the therapeutic effect of BCG	Interfere with clinical responce
	capreomycin	Increase neuromuscular—blocking effect of Aminoglycosides	Synergistic neuromuscular—blocking activity
	Cephalosporins (cefamandole, cefazolin, cefoperazone, cefotaxime,, cefotetan, cefoxitin, ceftazidime, ceftizoxime, ceftriaxone, cefuroxime, cephalothin,	Increased risk of Aminoglycosides nephrotoxicity	Synergistic nephrotoxicity. cephalosporins may spuriously elevate creatinine concentrations

DRUG	DRUG INTERACTION	EFFECT	MECHANISM OF INTERACTION
	cephapirin, cephradine)		
	clindamycin	Increased risk of Aminoglycosides nephrotoxicity	Synergistic nephrotoxicity
	cisplatin	Increased risk of Aminoglycosides nephrotoxicity	Both cisplatin and aminoglycosides have been reported to cause renal magnesium wasting. The exact mechanism of the interaction is unknown.
	colistimethate	Increase nephrotoxicity and neuromuscular—blocking effect of colistimethate	Synergistic nephrotoxicity and neuromuscular—blocking activity
	Digoxin	Decreased concentrations of digoxin.	Only with oral aminoglycosides that decrease absorption of digoxin
	Loop Diuretics [bumetanide furosemide, torsemide ethacrynic acid,	Increased risk of auditory toxicity and nephrotoxicity.	Loop Diuretics decrease Aminoglycosides clearance. Increase accumulation of

DRUG	DRUG INTERACTION	EFFECT	MECHANISM OF INTERACTION
			Aminoglycosides in renal tissues
	Penicillins [ampicillin methicillin, mezlocillin, nafcillin, oxacillin, penicillin G, piperacillin, ticarcillin]	Decrease in aminoglycoside activity	Inactivation of aminoglycoside.if mixed in same solution
	NSAIDs [diclofenac, etodolac, fenoprofen, flubiprofen, ibuprofen, indomethacin, ketoprofen, ketorolac, meclofenamate, mefenamic acid, nabumetone, naproxen, piroxicam, sulindac, tolmetin]	Increased concentrations of aminoglycoside in premature infants.	NSAIDs inhibit cyclooxygenase (COX), an enzyme involved in renal prostaglandin synthesis. This inhibition cause deterioration of glomerular filtration rate

Penicillins: Amoxicillin, Ampicillin, Bacampicillin, Carbenicillin, Cloxacillin, Dicloxacillin, Methicillin, Mezlocillin, Penicillin G, Penicillin V, Piperacillin, Ticarcillin

DRUG	DRUG INTERACTION	EFFECT	MECHANISM OF INTERACTION
Penicillins-class	Aminoglycosides	Decrease in aminoglycoside activity	Inactivation of aminoglycoside.if mixed in same solution
	BCG	Decrease the therapeutic effect of BCG	Interfere with clinical responce
	Fusidic acid	Decrease the therapeutic effect of penicillins	Fusidic acid inhibits protein synthesis, penicillins required active cell growth to be effective
	Mycophenolate	Penicillin decrease serum concentration of the active metabolites of mycophenolate	Impaired enterohepatic recirculation
	Methotrexate	Increased concentrations of methotrexate. Increased risk of methotrexate toxicity.	Penicillins are weak acids that compate with methotrexate for excretion sites in the renal tubules
	Oral contraceptive	Diminish the therapeutic effect	Penicillins reduce gut bacteria which

DRUG	DRUG INTERACTION	EFFECT	MECHANISM OF INTERACTION
	(estrogens)	of oral contraceptive (estrogens)	are important for hydrolysis of conjucated estrogen
	Tetracyclines[de meclocycline, doxycycline, minocycline, oxytetracycline, tetracycline]	Decreased effects of penicillins.	Antagonism of effect of bacteriostatic doxycyclin on bacteriocidal penicillins
	Warfarin	Increased effects of warfarin with large doses of IV penicillin. Nafcillin and dicloxacillin can caus ewarfarin resistance.	Not understood. The nafcillin-warfarin interaction is possibly due to increase in the metabolism of warfarin by the liver. Changes in bleeding times caused by the other penicillins appear to result from changes in antithrombin III activity, blood platelet changes and alterations in the fibrinogen-fibrin conversion. Dicloxacillin possibly reduces serum warfarin levels.
	Allopurinol	Increased rate of	Potentiation of

DRUG	DRUG INTERACTION	EFFECT	MECHANISM OF INTERACTION
		ampicillin-associated skin rash.	Ampicillin effect (not well defined)
	Atenolol	Decreased effects of atenolol.	due to impaired gastrointestinal absorption in the presence of ampicillin.

Cephalosporins: Cefamandole, Cefazolin, Cefonicid, Cefoperazone, Cefotaxime, Cefotetan, Cefoxitin, Ceftazidime, Ceftizoxime, Ceftriaxone, Cefuroxime, Cephalothin, Cephradine

DRUG	DRUG INTERACTION	EFFECT	MECHANISM OF INTERACTION
Cephalosporins	Aminoglycosides	Increased risk of Aminoglycosides nephrotoxicity	Synergistic nephrotoxicity. cephalosporins may spuriously elevate creatinine concentrations
	Antacids [aluminum hydroxide, aluminum-magnesium hydroxide, magnesium hydroxide, sodium bicarbonate]	Decrease absorption of cephalosporins	formation of Chelate between cephalosporins and antiacids

DRUG	DRUG INTERACTION	EFFECT	MECHANISM OF INTERACTION
	Warfarin	Increased effects of warfarin.	Cephalosporin – associated platelet inhibition.

Decrease in gastric normal flora that serve as aminor source of vit. K2 |
| | Uricosuric agents (probenecid, sulfinpyrazone | Decrease excretion of cephalosporins | Uricosuric agents compate for renal tubular excretion |
| Cefamandol,Cef onicid, Cefoperazone, Ceforanide, Cefotetan, Moxalactam

(See also Cephalosporin) | Ethanol | Disulfuram-like reaction. | These agents contain an N-methylthiotetrazol e (NMTT) side chain that may inhibit aldehyde dehydrogenase (ALDH) similar to disulfiram. Following ingestion of alcohol, inhibition of ALDH results in increased concentration of acetaldehyde, the accumulation of which produces an unpleasant physiologic response referred to as the 'disulfiram reaction. |
| Cephalexin | metformin | Cephalexin may | Impaired renal |

DRUG	DRUG INTERACTION	EFFECT	MECHANISM OF INTERACTION
(See also Cephalosporin)		increase serum concentration of metformin	clearance of metformin by cephalexin (competitive inhibitors)

Macrolide: Azithromycin, Clarithromycin, Erythromycin, Troleandomycin

DRUG	DRUG INTERACTION	EFFECT	MECHANISM OF INTERACTION
Macrolide	Cyclosporine	Increased concentrationsof cyclosporine.	Inhibition of CYP isoenzyme responsible for cyclosporine metabolism
	calcium channel blocker (amlodipine, diltiazem, isradipine, felodipine, nicardipine, nifedipine, verapamil)	increase serum concentration of calcium channel blocker, increase risk of fatigue, dizziness, bradycardia, hypotension	Inhibition of CYP3A4 by macrolides
	Corticosteroids (Betamethason, Corticotropin, Cortisone, Cosyntropin, Dexamethason,	Increased therapeutic/ toxic effects of corticosteroides.	inhibition of CYP3A4 by erythromycin

DRUG	DRUG INTERACTION	EFFECT	MECHANISM OF INTERACTION
	Fludrocortisone, Hydrocortisone, Methylprednisolone, Prednisolone, Prednisone, Triamcinolone)		
	digoxin	Increased concentrations/ toxic effect of digoxin.	Macrolide Antibiotics inhibit intestina and renal p-glycoprotein. Also macrolide might eradicate normal flora (ie. Eubacterium Lentum) that degrade some digoxin prior absorption, thus leaving greater quantity to be absorbed
	HMG-CoA Reductase Inhibitors	Increased risk of severemyopathy and rhabdomyolysis. [Exceptions: fluvastatin, pravastatin]	Inhibition of CYP3A4 mediated metabolism (simvastatin, lovastatin, atorvastatin)
	tacrolimus	Increased concentrations of tacrolimus.	inhibition of CYP3A4 by macrolides

DRUG	DRUG INTERACTION	EFFECT	MECHANISM OF INTERACTION
	Theophylline	Increased concentrations of theophylline.	Macrolide inhibit CYP3A4 isoenzymes.
	Quinolones, gatifloxacin, moxifloxacin, sparfloxacin	Increased risk of cardiac arrhythmias	Enhance the QTc-prolongation for each other
Clarithromycin *(See also macrolides)*	alfuzosin	Increase serum concentration of alfuzosin	Clarithromycin is CYP3A4 inhibitors, Alfuzosin metabolism by CYP3A4
	alfentanil	Increase serum concentration of alfentanil	inhibition of CYP3A4 by Clarithromycin
	almotriptan	Increase serum concentration of almotriptan	inhibition of CYP3A4 by Clarithromycin
	Antifungal agents (azole derivatives, systemic)	Increase serum concentration of Clarithromycin(QTc-prolongation) and serum concentration of Antifungal agents	inhibition of CYP3A4 by Clarithromycin and azole derivatives

DRUG	DRUG INTERACTION	EFFECT	MECHANISM OF INTERACTION
	Antineoplastic agents (vinca alkaloids)	Increase serum concentration of vinca alkaloids, also increase the distribution of alkaloids into certain cell and/or tissue. High incidence of grade 4 neutropenia	inhibition of CYP3A4 by Clarithromycin, and p-glycoprotien – mediated alkaloide transport
	buspirone.	Increased effects of buspirone.	CYP3A4 inhibition by clarithromycine
	Benzodiazepines (metabolized by oxidation)(except ion for lorazepam, oxazepam and temazepam)	Increase serum concentration of Benzodiazepines Prolonged sedation and respiratory depression.	inhibition of CYP3A4 by Clarithromycin
	Bromocriptine	Increased concentrations of bromocriptine.	inhibition of CYP isoenzymes by Clarithromycin
	Carbamazepine	Increased concentrations of carbamazepine.	Inhibition of hepatic metabolism of carbamazepine by inhibition of CYP3A4 enzymes
	Cisapride	Increase concentration of cisapride lead to	Inhibit the CYP isoenzyme metabolisim of

DRUG	DRUG INTERACTION	EFFECT	MECHANISM OF INTERACTION
		cardiac conduction abnormality	cisapride
	Calcium channel blockers (diltiazem, felodipine, isradipine, nifedipine,nicardipine, nislodipine,nitredipine, verapamil	Increase serum concentration of Calcium channel blockers	inhibition of CYP3A4 by Clarithromycin
	colchicine	Increase serum concentration of colchicines. Colchicines toxicity (gastrointestinal symptoms, hematological abnormalities,neuropathies, myopathies	inhibition of CYP3A4 by Clarithromycin, and p-glycoprotien – mediated colchicine transport
	Corticosteroids	Increase serum concentration of Corticosteroids. Increase signs and symptoms of corticosteroids toxicity	inhibition of CYP3A4 by Clarithromycin
	clopidogrel	Diminish the therapeutic effect of clopidogrel	CYP3A4 inhibition of

DRUG	DRUG INTERACTION	EFFECT	MECHANISM OF INTERACTION
			by Clarithromycin cause reduction in clopidogrel bioactivation
	Dihydroergotamine	Increase serum concentration of Dihydroergotamine	inhibition of CYP3A4 by Clarithromycin
	disopyramide	Enhance QTc-prolongation of disopyramide, increase concentration of disopyramide	inhibition of CYP3A4 by Clarithromycin
	Eplerenone	Increase serum concentration of eplerenone	inhibition of CYP3A4 by Clarithromycin
	Ergot	Acute ergotism (peripheral ischemia).	inhibition of CYP3A4 by Clarithromycin
	pimozide	Enhance QTc-prolongation of pimozide, increase concentration of pimozide	inhibition of CYP3A4 by Clarithromycin
	Phosphodiasterase 5	Increase serum concentration of	inhibition of

DRUG	DRUG INTERACTION	EFFECT	MECHANISM OF INTERACTION
	inhibitors(sildenafil, tasalafil, vaedenafil)	(sildenafil, tasalafil, vaedenafil), and potential increase of side effects	CYP3A4 by Clarithromycin
	Quinine	Increase risk of elevated quinine serum level and potential adverse cardiac effects and QTc-prolongation of quinine	The precise mechanism is unknown, but likely result from inhibition of quinine metabolisim by CYP3A4 inhibitors
	Rifamycins	Increased rifamycin adverse effects (elevated hepatic enzymes, leucopenia, thrombocytopenia)	inhibition of CYP3A4 by Clarithromycin
	salmeterol	Increase serum concentration of salmeterol	inhibition of CYP3A4 by Clarithromycin
	tamsulosin	Increase serum concentration of tamsulosin	inhibition of CYP3A4 by Clarithromycin
	thioridazine	Enhance QTc-prolongation of thioridazine	inhibition of CYP3A4 by Clarithromycin

DRUG	DRUG INTERACTION	EFFECT	MECHANISM OF INTERACTION
	Warfarin	Increased effects of warfarin (bleeding tendency).	inhibition of CYP3A4 by Clarithromycin
	zidovudine	Enhance the myelosuppressive effect of zidovudine. Evidence of greater hepatotoxicity (decrease erythrocytes, neutrophils, and lymphocyte)	Absorption mediated interaction
Erythromycin *(See also macrolides)*	alfentanil	Increase serum concentration of alfentanil	inhibition of CYP3A4 by erythromycin
	Antifungal agents (azole derivatives, systemic)	Increase serum concentration of Clarithromycin(QTc-prolongation) and serum concentration of Antifungal agents	inhibition of CYP3A4 by erythromycin and azole derivatives
	Benzodiazepines	Increased concentrations of	inhibition of

DRUG	DRUG INTERACTION	EFFECT	MECHANISM OF INTERACTION
		benzodiazepine. Prolonged sedation and respiratory depression.	CYP3A4 by erythromycin
	Bromocriptine	Increased concentrations of bromocriptine.	inhibition of CYP isoenzymes by erythromycin
	Buspirone	Increased effects of buspirone	CYP3A4 inhibition by erythromycin
	colchicine	Increase serum concentration of colchicines. Colchicines toxicity (gastrointestinal symptoms, hematological abnormalities,neuropathies, myopathies	inhibition of CYP3A4 by erythromycin, and p-glycoprotien – mediated colchicine transport
	Calcium channel blockers(diltiazem, felodipine, isradipine, nifedipine, nicardipine, nislodipine, nitredipine verapamil	Increase serum concentration of Calcium channel blockers	inhibition of CYP3A4 by erythromycin
	Carbamazepine	Increased concentrations of	Inhibition of hepatic metabolism

DRUG	DRUG INTERACTION	EFFECT	MECHANISM OF INTERACTION
		carbamazepine.	of carbamazepine and inhibition of CYP3A4 enzymes
	disopyramide	Enhance QTc-prolongation of disopyramide, increase concentration of disopyramide	inhibition of CYP3A4 by erythromycin
	Ergot	Acute ergotism (peripheral ischemia).	inhibition of CYP3A4 by erythromycin
	pimozide	Enhance QTc-prolongation of pimozide, increase concentration of pimozide	inhibition of CYP3A4 by erythromycin
	Rifamycins	Increased rifamycin adverse effects (elevated hepatic enzymes, leucopenia, thrombocytopenia)	inhibition of CYP3A4 by erythromycin
	tetrabenazine	QTc-prolongation of tetrabenazine	inhibition of CYP2D6 by erythromycin
	thioridazine	Enhance QTc-prolongation of	inhibition of

DRUG	DRUG INTERACTION	EFFECT	MECHANISM OF INTERACTION
		thioridazine	CYP3A4 by erythromycin
	Warfarin	Increased effects of warfarin (bleeding tendency).	inhibition of CYP3A4 by erythromycin

Quinolones: Ciprofloxacin, Gatifloxacin, Gemifloxacin, Levofloxacin, Moxifloxacin, Nalidixic Acid, Norfloxacin, Ofloxacin, Sparfloxacin, Trovafloxacin

DRUG	DRUG INTERACTION	EFFECT	MECHANISM OF INTERACTION
Quinolones	Iron(Oral) [ferrous fumarate, ferrousgluconate, ferrous sulfate, iron polysaccharide]	Decreased GI absorption of quinolone.	Formation of insoluble complex between the antibiotic and iron ion
	Antacids[aluminum hydroxide, aluminum-magnesium hydroxide, calcium acetate, calcium carbonate, magnesium hydroxide]	Decreased GI absorption of quinolone.	The carbonyl and 4-oxo functional groups on the antibiotics forms a chelate with cations of the antiacid

DRUG	DRUG INTERACTION	EFFECT	MECHANISM OF INTERACTION
	Corticosteroids	Increase serum concentration of Corticosteroids. Increase signs and symptoms of corticosteroids toxicity	inhibition of CYP3A4
	insulin	Hypoglycemia 1-2 days of initiating quinolone therapy. Hypoglycemia tend to occur later in therapy lend	Insulin may simply enhance the insulin-secreting effect of quinolone
	Macrolide antibiotics (clarithromycin, erythromycin, telithromycin)	Increased risk of cardiac arrhythmias	Enhance the QTc-prolongation for each other
	Nonsteroidal anti-inflammatory agents	Enhance the neuroexcitatory and/or seizure-potentiating effect of quinolone	In vitro and in vivo animal data describe enhanced central GABA-A inhibition as a plausible mechanism of such interaction
	Sucralfate	Decreased GI absorption of quinolone.	Formation of insoluble complex between aluminium of sucralfate and quinolone

DRUG	DRUG INTERACTION	EFFECT	MECHANISM OF INTERACTION
	sulfonylureas	Quinolone enhance the hypoglycemic effect of sulfonylureas (early in the course of administration) Quinolones diminish sulfonylureas hypoglycemic effect in long-term combination	Quinolones have dual effects on pancreatic islet cell, initially stimulate insulin release ,but inhibiting insulin release after long—term
	Theophylline	Increased concentrations of theophylline.	Quinolones inhibit CYP1A2 and/or CYP3A4, mediated theophylline metabolism
	quinapril	Decreased GI absorption of quinolone.	Chelation of the magnesium ion that are part of quinapril formulation and quinolone
	warfarin	Increase effect of warfarin	In vitro evidence, quinolones are able to diplace warfarin from protein binding site
	Zinc salts	Decreased GI absorption of	Formation of insoluble complex

DRUG	DRUG INTERACTION	EFFECT	MECHANISM OF INTERACTION
		quinolone.	
Nalidixic Acid *(See also quinolones)*	warfarin	Increased effects of warfarin.	In vitro evidence, Nalidixic Acid is able to diplace warfarin from protein binding site
Ciprofloxacin, Norfloxacin *(See also quinolones)*	Cyclosporine	Increased risk of nephrotoxicity.	Inhibition of CYP3A4
	caffeine	Decrease the metabolism of caffeine	Inhibition of CYP1A2
	Food [milk]	Decreased GI absorption of ciprofloxacin.	The carbonyl and 4-oxo functional groups on the antibiotics forms a chelate with cations of the calcium salts
	methotrexate	Increased serum concentrations of methotrexate	Delay in methotrexate elimination. The exact mechanism is unclear
	phenytoin	Decrease serum concentration of phenytoin.

Patient experience seizure | The mechanism is unclear.

Animal data indicate change in renal excretion of |

DRUG	DRUG INTERACTION	EFFECT	MECHANISM OF INTERACTION
			phenytoin. Ciprofloxacin alone can cause seizure
Ofloxacin (See also quinolones)	Procainamide	Increased concentrations of procainamide.	Competition for the excretion site in the kidney
gatifloxacin, moxifloxacin, sparfloxacin (See also quinolones)	Amiodarone	Increased risk of cardiac arrhythmias	Enhance the QTc-prolongatoion for each drug
	Disopyramide	Increased risk of cardiac arrhythmias	Enhance the QTc-prolongatoion for each drug.
	Phenothiazines	Increased risk of cardiac arrhythmias	Enhance the QTc-prolongatoion for each drug.
	Procainamide	Increased risk of cardiac arrhythmias	Enhance the QTc-prolongatoion for each drug.
	Quinidine	Increased risk of cardiac arrhythmias	Enhance the QTc-prolongatoion for each drug.
	Sotalol	Increased effects of beta—blocker	Enhance the QTc-prolongatoion for each drug.

DRUG	DRUG INTERACTION	EFFECT	MECHANISM OF INTERACTION
	Tricyclic Antidepressants [amitriptyline, desipramine, doxepin, imipramine, nortriptyline]	Increased risk of cardiac arrhythmias	Enhance the QTc-prolongatoion for each drug.

Tetracyclines: Demeclocycline, Doxycycline, Methacycline, Minocycline, Oxytetracycline, Tetracycline

DRUG	DRUG INTERACTION	EFFECT	MECHANISM OF INTERACTION
Tetracyclines	Antacids[aluminum hydroxide, aluminum-magnesium hydroxide, calcium acetate, calcium carbonate, magnesium hydroxide]	Decreased GI absorption of tetracycline.	formation of Chelate between tetracycline and antiacids
	atovaquone	Decrease serum concentration of atovaquone (40%)	unclear
	BCG	Decrease the therapeutic effect of BCG	Interfere with clinical responce
	Bismuth Salts	Decrease serum concentration of	Decreased GI absorption of

DRUG	DRUG INTERACTION	EFFECT	MECHANISM OF INTERACTION
		tetracyclines.	tetracycline,chelation
	Bile acid sequestrant (cholestyramine, colesevelam, colestipol	Decrease absorption of tetracyclines	Colestipol bind to tetracycline in GIT. The mechanism of other bile acid sequestrant is unknown
	colchicine	Increase serum concentration of colchicines	Tetracycline is moderate CYP3A4 inhibitor
	digoxin	Increased concentrations of digoxin.	tetracyclines reduces gut flora that would metabolize some digoxin prior the absorption
	eplerenone	Increase serum concentration of eplerenon	Tetracycline is moderate CYP3A4 inhibitor
	fentanyl	Increase serum concentration of fentanyl	Tetracycline is moderate CYP3A4 inhibitor
	Iron Salts (Oral) [ferrousfumarate, ferrous gluconate, ferrous sulfate	Decrease serum concentration of tetracycline	Decreased GI absorptionof tetracycline, chelation between tetracycline and iron in GIT.
	methotrexate	Increase serum	suppressing

DRUG	DRUG INTERACTION	EFFECT	MECHANISM OF INTERACTION
		concentration of methotrexate.	metabolism of the drug by bacteria in GIT
	Penicillins	Diminish the therapeutic effect of penicillin	Antagonism of effect of bacteriostatic doxycyclin on bacteriocidal penicillins
	Retinoic acid derivative	Tetracycline may enhance the toxic /adrerse effect of retinoic acid derivative{development of pseudomotor cerebri (intracranial hypertension)}	The mechanism is unclear, but may result from each agent ability to independently increase intracranial pressure
	sucralfate	Decrease GIT absorption of tetracyclines	Binding of the amide and/or amine groupe of tetracycline molecule to aluminum moieties of sucralfate
	Urinary Alkalinizers [potassium citrate, sodium acetate, sodium bicarbonate, sodium citrate, sodium lactate, tromethamine]	Decreased concentrations of tetracycline.	formation of Chelate between tetracycline and Urinary Alkalinizers. Increase excretion of tetracyclines

DRUG	DRUG INTERACTION	EFFECT	MECHANISM OF INTERACTION
	zinc gluconate, zinc sulfate	Decreased GI absorption of tetracycline.	Formation of relatively insoluble chelate in GIT.
	quinapril	Decreased GI absorption of tetracycline.	Chelation of the magnesium ion that are part of quinapril formulation and tetracycline
Doxycycline *(See also* tetracyclines*)*	Barbiturates	Decreased concentrations of doxycycline.	Incuction of metabolism or excretion of doxycycline by barbiturates (enzymes and/ or transports is uncertain)
	Carbamazepine	Decreased concentrations of doxycycline.	Incuction of metabolism or excretion of doxycycline by barbiturates (enzymes and/ or transports is uncertain)
	phenytoin	Decreased concentrations of doxycycline.	Incuction of metabolism or excretion of doxycycline by barbiturates (enzymes and/ or transports is uncertain)

DRUG	DRUG INTERACTION	EFFECT	MECHANISM OF INTERACTION
	Rifamycins: rifabutin, rifampin	Decreased concentrations of doxycycline.	increase the clearance of doxycycline when coadministered

Chloramphenicol

DRUG	DRUG INTERACTION	EFFECT	MECHANISM OF INTERACTION
Chloramphenic ol	barbiturates	chloramphenicol Increase serum concentration of barbiturates. Barbiturates decrease serum concentration of chloramphinicol	Chloramphenicol diminish barbiturates metabolism. Barbiturates inhibit CYP isoenzymes responsible for chloramphenicol metabolism
	cyanocobalamin	Decrease therapeutic effect of cyanocobalamin	Chloramphenicol interrupted red blood cell maturation
	Iron Products,	reduce the therapeutic efficacy of iron for the treatment of anaemia	decreasing erythropoiesis due to direct bone marrow depression
	Phenytoin	Increased concentrations of phenytoin(three	Chloramphenicol inhibit the metabolism of

DRUG	DRUG INTERACTION	EFFECT	MECHANISM OF INTERACTION
		fold). Variable effects on concentrations of chloramphenicol.	phenytoin.
	refampin	Decrease serum concentration of chloramphinicol	Induction of CYP2b responsible for metabolism of chloramphenicol
	Sulfonylureas	Increased hypoglycemic effects of sulfonylurea.	Unclear, possibly due to inhibition of sulfonylurea metabolism
	Warfarin	Increased effects of warfarin.	Chloramphenicol inhibit the metabolism of phenytoin.

Clindamycin

DRUG	DRUG INTERACTION	EFFECT	MECHANISM OF INTERACTION
Clindamycin	Aluminum Salts [aluminum carbonate, aluminum hydroxide, aluminum phosphate, attapulgite, kaolin, magaldrate]	Delayed GI absorption of clindamycin.	formation of Chelate between clindamycin and antiacids
	Aminoglycosides	Increased risk of	Synergistic

DRUG	DRUG INTERACTION	EFFECT	MECHANISM OF INTERACTION
		Aminoglycosides nephrotoxicity	nephrotoxicity
	mycophenolate	Decrease serum conc.of active metabolite of mycophenolate	Clindamycin kill glucuronidase—producing bacteria in GIT that mediate the metabolism of mycophenolate

Dapsone

DRUG	DRUG INTERACTION	EFFECT	MECHANISM OF INTERACTION
Dapsone	rifamycin derivatives	decrease serum concentration of dapsone	induction of CYP3A4 enzyme by rifamycin
	Trimethoprim	Increased concentrations of both drugs	unknown
	urecosuric agents (probenecid, sulfinpyrazone)	increase serum concentration of dapson	inhibition of urinary excretion of dapson

Metronidazole

DRUG	DRUG INTERACTION	EFFECT	MECHANISM OF INTERACTION
Metronidazole	amprenavir	Enhanced	Inhibition of

DRUG	DRUG INTERACTION	EFFECT	MECHANISM OF INTERACTION
		toxicity/ adverse effect of amprevie	propylene glycol metabolism (CYP3A4 inhibitor) in the formulation of amprenavir
	busulfan	Increase serum concentration of busulfan	unclear
	Barbiturates [amobarbital, aprobarbital, butabarbital butalbital, mephobarbital, pentobarbital, phenobarbital]	Therapeutic failure of metronidazole.	Increase Metronidazole elimination (metabolism of Metronidazole ont affected
	colchicine	Increase serum concentration (increase toxic effect)	CYP3A4 inhibition by mtronidazole
	Disulfiram	Acute psychosis or confusion.	unknown
	eplerenone	Increase serum concentration of eplerenone	CYP3A4 inhibition by mtronidazole
	everolimus	Increase AUC of everolimus by 2-3 fold	CYP3A4 inhibition by mtronidazole
	Ethanol	Disulfiram-like reaction.	Inhibition of acetaldehyde

DRUG	DRUG INTERACTION	EFFECT	MECHANISM OF INTERACTION
			dehydrogenase by metronidazol
	mebendazole	Increase toxic effect of metronidazole (high risk of stevens—Johnson syndrum or toxic epidermal necrolysis	unclear
	mycophenolate	Decrease serum concentration of mycophenolate (decrease effectiveness)	Inhibition of active metabolite formation of mycophenolate
	phenytoin	Metronidazole increase concentration of phenytoin, phenytoin decrease serum concentration of metronidazol	Metronidazole inhibit one or more of the enzymes responsible for phenytoin metabolism, phenytoin induce metronidazole metabolism
	salmeterol	Increase cardiovascular adverse effect (increase heart rate, prolonged QT interval,..ect) of salmeterol	Inhibition of CYP3A4 by metronidazol
	Vitamin K	Increase	Metronidazol

DRUG	DRUG INTERACTION	EFFECT	MECHANISM OF INTERACTION
	antagonists	prothrombin time	apparently inhibit CYP2C9 ,the isoenzyme responsible for S-warfarin metabolism

Trimethoprim/ Sulfamethoxazole

DRUG	DRUG INTERACTION	EFFECT	MECHANISM OF INTERACTION
Trimethoprim/ Sulfamethoxazole	ACE inhibitors	Trimethoprim enhance the hyperkalemic effect of ACE inhibitors	Both drug reduce renal potassium excretion
	Angiotensin II receptor blockers	Trimethoprim enhance the hyperkalemic effect of Angiotensin II receptor blockers	Both drug reduce renal potassium excretion
	Cyclosporine	Decreased effects of cyclosporine. Increased risk of nephrotoxicity with oral sulfonamides.	unknown
	Dapsone	Increased concentrations of both drugs.	unknown

DRUG	DRUG INTERACTION	EFFECT	MECHANISM OF INTERACTION
	methenamine	Enhance the adverse/toxic effect of sulphonamide derivatives	formation of insoluble precipitate in urine that prevent the formation of formaldehyde
	Methotrexate	Increased risk of bone marrow suppression and megaloblastic anemia.	Both drug cause folate deficiency (suppression of dihydrofolate reductase)
	Phenytoin	Increased concentrations of phenytoin.	Inhibition of CYP isoenzymes by Trimethoprim
	Procainamide	Increased concentrations of procainamide	Competition for the excretion site in the renal tubules
	Sulfonylureas	Enhance the hypoglycemic effect of sulfonylurea. Exception: Glyburide	Inhibition of Sulfonylureas metabolism by sulfonamides. Displacement of Sulfonylureas from plasma protein binding site

Vancomycin

DRUG	DRUG INTERACTION	EFFECT	MECHANISM OF INTERACTION
Vancomycin	atracurium, gallamine triethiodide, pancuronium, pipecuronium, tubocurarine, vecuronium	Increased effects of nondepolarizing muscle relaxant (prolonged respiratory depression).	unknown
	Nonsteroidal anti-inflammatory drugs	Increase toxic/adverse effect of vancomycin	unknown

ANTIMYCOBACTERIAL AGENTS

DRUG	DRUG INTERACTION	EFFECT	MECHANISM OF INTERACTION
Isoniazid	Carbamazepine	Increased risk of carbamazepine toxicity	Inhibition of CYP isoenzymes mediated carbamazepine metabolism by Isoniazid.
	clopidogrel	Decrease serum concentration of active metabolite of clobidogrel	Inhibition of CYP2C19 by INH
	eplerenon	Increase serum concentration of eplerenon	Inhibition of CYP3A4 by INH

	phenytoin	Increased concentrations of phenytoin.	Isoniazid inhibit CYP2C19, CYP2C9 and CYP3A4 mediated phenytoin metabolism

Rifamycins: Rifabutin, Rifampin, Rifapentine

DRUG	DRUG INTERACTION	EFFECT	MECHANISM OF INTERACTION
Rifamycins	Acetaminophen	Decrease serum concentration of Acetaminophen	Induction of glucuronidation of acetaminophen (ie. Detoxification) pathway
	Antiemetics(5HT3 antagonists) alosetron, ondansetron	Decrease serum concentration of Antiemetics(5HT3 antagonists)	unknown
	Azole Antifungals	Decreased concentrations of azole antifungal. Increase serum concentration of rifamycin	Induction of CYP3A4 by rifamycin. Inhibition of CYP isoenzymes by azole antifungal.
	barbiturate	Rifampin may decrease the plasma concentrations of barbiturates	inducing hepatic metabolism by Rifampin
	beta-blocker	Decreased effects of	Induction of

DRUG	DRUG INTERACTION	EFFECT	MECHANISM OF INTERACTION
	(atenolol, bisoprolol, metoprolol, propranolol)	beta-blocker.	CYP3A4 isoenzyme by Rifamycins
	Buspirone	Decreased buspirone effects	Induction of CYP3A4 isoenzyme by Rifamycins
	Calcium channel blockers	Decrease therapeutic effect of Calcium channel blockers	Induction of CYP3A4 isoenzymes, especially in the intestinal mucosa.(inhibit metabolism and absorption)
	chloramphenicol	Increase metabolism of chloramphinicol	Induction of CYP2B by rifamycins
	Clarithromycin	Increased rifamycin adverse effects (elevated hepatic enzymes, leucopenia, thrombocytopenia)	inhibition of CYP3A4 by Clarithromycin
	clopidogrel	Enhance the therapeutic effects of clopidogrel	CYP3A4 induction cause increase in clopidogrel bioactivation
	Contraceptives (progestins, estrogens)	Contraceptive failure	Induction of hormone metabolism by rifamycin

DRUG	DRUG INTERACTION	EFFECT	MECHANISM OF INTERACTION
	Corticosteroids	Decreased effects of corticosteroid.	Induction of CYP isoenzymes by rifamycins
	Cyclosporine	Decreased concentrations of cyclosporine.	Induction of CYP3A4 by rifamycins
	disopyramide	Decrease serum concentration of disopyramide	Induction of CYP3A4 isoenzymes
	delavirdine	Decreased concentrationsof delavirdine	CYP3A4 induction by rifampin
	Doxycycline	Decreased concentrations of doxycycline.	increase the clearance of doxycycline when coadministered
	Erythromycin	Increased rifamycin adverse effects (elevated hepatic enzymes, leucopenia, thrombocytopenia)	inhibition of CYP3A4 by erythromycin
	Estrogens	Decreased concentrations of estrogen	Induction of CYP3A4 by rifamycins
	Haloperidol	Decreased effects of haloperidol.	Induction of CYP3A4 by rifamycins

DRUG	DRUG INTERACTION	EFFECT	MECHANISM OF INTERACTION
	HMG-CoA Reductase Inhibitors,	Decreased effects of statin. [Exception: pravastatin]	Induction of CYP3A4 by rifamycins
	indinavir	Decreased concentrations of in dinavir. Increased concentrations of rifamycin.	Induction of metabolism and elimination of dinavir by Rifamycins. CYP3A4 inhibition by indinavir
	Methadone	Decreased effects of methadone. Possible with—drawal symptoms in patients on chronic methadone therapy.	Induction of CYP2B6, CYP2C9, CYP3A4 mediated methadone metabolism by rifampin
	Morphine	Decreased analgesic effects of morphine.	Induction of CYP3A4 and CYP2C8 by rifampin
	mycophenolate	Decrease the serum concentration (2-fold) of active metabolites of mycophenolate	Increase glucuronidation of MPA and decrease biliary excretion of MPA glucuronides
	Nelfinavir	Decreased concentrations of nelfinavir.	CYP3A4 induction by rifampin
	Phenytoin	Decreased concentrations of	CYP isoenzyme induction of

DRUG	DRUG INTERACTION	EFFECT	MECHANISM OF INTERACTION
		phenytoin.	rifamycins
	Quinidine	Decreased concentrations/ effect of quinidine.	Induction of CYP3A4. Protein displacement of quinidine and increase clearance and metabolism quinidine
	Quinine	Decreased concentrations of quinine.	Protein displacement of Quinine and increase clearance and metabolism Quinine
	Ritonavir	Decreased concentrations of ritonavir. Increased concentrations of rifabutin.	CYP3A4 induction by rifampin
	Sulfonylureas	Decreased concentrations of sulfonylurea.	Induction of CYP2C9 by rifamycins
	tamoxifen	Decrease therapeutic effect of tamoxifen	Induction of CYP3A4 isoenzymes by rifamycins
	Tacrolimus	Decreased concentrations of tacrolimus.	CYP3A4 induction by rifamycins
	Theophyllines	Decreased	CYP3A4 and

DRUG	DRUG INTERACTION	EFFECT	MECHANISM OF INTERACTION
		concentrations of theophylline.	CYP1A2 induction by rifamycins
	Tricyclic Antidepressants	Decreased therapeutic effects of tricyclic antidepressant.	Induction of CYP isoenzymes by rifamycins
	Valproic acid	Decrease serum concentration of valproic acid	CYP2C19 and CYP2C9 induction of rifamycins
	Warfarin	Decreased effects of warfarin.	Induction of CYP isoenzymes by rifamycins
Rifampin *(See also rifamycins)*	atazanavir	Decrease serum concentration of atazanavir	CYP3A4 induction by rifampin
	Disopyramide	Decreased concentrations of disopyramide.	CYP3A4 induction by rifampin
	Isoniazid	Increased risk of hepatotoxicity.	Increase metabolism of Isoniazid to form hydrazine, an hepatotoxic metabolite

ANTIVIRAL AGENTS

DRUG	DRUG INTERACTION	EFFECT	MECHANISM OF INTERACTION
Protease Inhibitors [amprenavir, indinavir, nelfinavir, ritonavir, saquinavir]	amiodarone	Increased concentrations of amiodarone.	Potent inhibitionn of CYP3A4 by Protease Inhibitors
	Azole Antifungals [fluconazole, itraconazole, ketoconazole]	Increase serum concentration of protease inhibitors.	Inhibition of CYP3A4 by azol Antifungals additionally for itraconazole and ketoconazole to inhibite p-glycoprotein
	Benzodiazepines	Increased concentrations of benzodiazepine. Prolonged sedation and respiratory depression.	Inhibition of CYP3A4 and p-glycoprotein by indinavir that inhibit metabolism and transport of Benzodiazepines
	Ergot Alkaloids	Increased risk of ergot toxicity (peripheral ischemia, peripheral vasospasm).	Inhibition of CYP3A4 by Delavirdine that reduce ergot metabolism
	Estrogens [chlorotrianisene, conjugated estrogens,	Loss of contraceptive efficacyof ethinyl estradiol.	Unclear, but may related to enzyme induction of ritonavir

DRUG	DRUG INTERACTION	EFFECT	MECHANISM OF INTERACTION
	diethylstilbesterol, esterified estrogens, estradiol, estrone, estropipate, ethinyl estradiol, quinestrol]		
	flecainide	Increased concentrations of flecainide.	Potent inhibitionn of CYP3A4 by Protease Inhibitors
	quinidine	Increased concentrations/ toxic effect of quinidine (life-threatening adverse effect).	Potent CYP3A4 inhibitors of protease inhibitors decrease metabolism of quinidine
Acyclovir	cimetidine	increase serum concentration of acyclovir	Competition of the drugs for the renal tubule secretion sites
	Theophyllines	Increased concentrations of theophylline.	inhibition of theophylline oxidative metabolism

Delavirdine

DRUG	DRUG INTERACTION	EFFECT	MECHANISM OF INTERACTION
Delavirdine	alfuzocin	Increase serum concentration of alfuzocin	CYP3A4 inhibition by delavirdine
	clopidogrel	Decrease serum concentration of active metabolites of clopidogrel (decrease effectivity)	Inhibition of CYP2C19 mediated clopidogrel metabolism/ activation
	Ergot Alkaloids	Increased risk of ergot toxicity (peripheral ischemia, peripheral vasospasm).	Inhibition of CYP3A4 by Delavirdine that reduce ergot metabolism
	Rifamycins	Decreased concentrationsof delavirdine	CYP3A4 induction by rifampin
	salmeterol	Increase serum concentration of salmeterol	CYP3A4 inhibition by delavirdine
	tamoxifen	Reduce the clinical effectiveness of tamoxifen	CYP2D6 inhibition by delavirdine cause decrease in the concentration of highly antiestrogenic tamoxifen and 4-hydroxy-n-desmethyl-tamoxifen

DRUG	DRUG INTERACTION	EFFECT	MECHANISM OF INTERACTION
			(endoxifen)
	tamsulosin	Increase tamsulosin AUC (3 folds) and maximum serum concentration (2 folds)	CYP3A4 inhibition by delavirdine

Didanosine

DRUG	DRUG INTERACTION	EFFECT	MECHANISM OF INTERACTION
Didanosine	Alcohol (ethyl)	Enhance the adverse/toxic effect of didanosine specifically the risk of pancreatitis may be increase	Both have been independently associated with pancreatitis
	allopurinol	Increase risk of toxicity of didanosine	Inihibition of didanosine metabolism by inhibition of xanthine oxidase mediated metabolism, or indirectly by accumulation of hypoxanthine phosphorylase-mediated didanosin metabolism

DRUG	DRUG INTERACTION	EFFECT	MECHANISM OF INTERACTION
	indinavir	Decrase serum concentration of indinavir	Decrase in GIT absorption of indinavir caused by buffer mediated increase in gastric PH by Didanosine formulation
	itraconazole	Decreased GI absorption of itraconazole.	The buffer system of didanosine may reduce absorption of itraconazole by increasing gastric pH
	ketoconazole	Decreased GI absorption of ketoconazole.	The buffer system of didanosine may reduce absorption of ketoconazole by increasing gastric pH.
	Quinolones [gatifloxacin, moxifloxacin, sparfloxacin]	Decreased GI absorption of quinolone.	Formation of an insoluble chelates with the aluminum and magnesium ions that used as buffers in didanosine formulation

Ganciclovir

DRUG	DRUG INTERACTION	EFFECT	MECHANISM OF INTERACTION
Ganciclovir	Zidovudine	Increased risk of life-threatening hematologic toxicity.	due to additive myelosuppressive effects

Indinavir

DRUG	DRUG INTERACTION	EFFECT	MECHANISM OF INTERACTION
Indinavir (See also protease inhibitors)	alfuzosin	Increase serum concentration of alfuzosin	CYP3A4 inhibition by indinavir
	amiodarone	Increase serum concentration of amiodarone, cause serious/life-threatening adverse effects	CYP3A4 inhibition by indinavir
	Didanosine	Decreased serum concentration of indinavir.	Decrase in GIT absorption of indinavir caused by buffer mediated increase in gastric PH by Didanosine formulation

DRUG	DRUG INTERACTION	EFFECT	MECHANISM OF INTERACTION
	Ergot	Increased risk of ergot toxicity (peripheral ischemia, peripheral vasospasm).	CYP3A4 inhibition by indinavir
	quinidine	Increase risk of cardiovascular effects QTc prolongation, hypotension, angina, syncope and Cinchonism	CYP3A4 inhibition by indinavir
	Rifamycins [rifabutin, rifampin, rifapentine]	Decreased concentrations of in dinavir. Increased concentrations of rifamycin.	Induction of metabolism and elimination of dinavir by Rifamycins. CYP3A4 inhibition by indinavir
	salmeterol	Increase serum concentration of almeterol cause,headache, muscle pain,hypotension,	CYP3A4 inhibition by indinavir

Ritonavir

DRUG	DRUG INTERACTION	EFFECT	MECHANISM OF INTERACTION
Ritonavir	Amiodarone	Increased	CYP3A4 inhibitors

DRUG	DRUG INTERACTION	EFFECT	MECHANISM OF INTERACTION
(See also protease inhibitors)		concentrations of amiodarone.	by ritonavir
	Azole Antifungals[fluconazole, itraconazole, ketoconazole]	Increased concentrations of ritonavir. Ritonavir increase concentration of Azole	CYP3A4 and P-glycoprotein inhibition by Azol. CYP3A4 inhibition by ritonavir
	Buproprion	Decrase serum concentration of Buproprion (decrease effect) , increase concentration of active metabolite hydroxybupropion.	inhibition of CYP2C6 mediated—Buproprion metabolism by ritonavir
	Clozapine	Increased concentrations of clozapine.	Inhibition of CYP3A4 and p-glycoprotein by ritonavir that mediate metabolism and transport of Clozapine
	Ethinyl Estradiol	Loss of contraceptive efficacyof ethinyl estradiol.	involve ritonavir induction of glucuronosyltransferase and/or CYP450 hydroxylation. Since estrogens and progestins may

DRUG	DRUG INTERACTION	EFFECT	MECHANISM OF INTERACTION
			share common routes of metabolism
	Flecainide	Increased concentrations of flecainide case cardiac arrhythmias.	CYP2D6 inhibition by ritonavir
	pimozide	Increase risk of QTc prolongation and life threatening arrhythmias	Inhibition of CYP3A4 isoenzymes by ritonavir
	Meperidine	Decreased efficacy of meperidine and increased risk of neurologic toxicity.	induction of CYP2B6, CYP2C19 that metabolite Meperidine to highly toxic normeperidine
	Piroxicam	Increased risk of piroxicam toxicity.	Inhibition of CYP 2C9 by Ritonavir
	Propoxyphene	Increased risk of propoxyphene toxicity (seizures, respiratory depression, apnea, cardiac arrhythmias, pulmonary edema).	CYP3A4 inhibition by ritonavir
	salmeterol	Increase serum concentration of	CYP3A4 inhibition by ritonavir

DRUG	DRUG INTERACTION	EFFECT	MECHANISM OF INTERACTION
		almeterol cause,headache, muscle pain,hypotension	

Zidovudine

DRUG	DRUG INTERACTION	EFFECT	MECHANISM OF INTERACTION
Zidovudine	clarithromycin	Enhance the myelosuppressive effect of zidovudine. Evidence of greater hepatotoxicity (decrease erythrocytes, neutrophils, and lymphocyte)	Absorption mediated interaction
	Ganciclovir	Increased risk of life-threatening hematologic toxicity.	due to additive myelosuppressive effects
	Probenecid	Rash, malaise, myalgia, and fever.	Probenecid reduce the metabolism (glucuronidation of zidovudine in liver

Azole Antifungals: *Fluconazole, Itraconazole, Ketoconazole, Miconazole, Voriconazole*

DRUG	DRUG INTERACTION	EFFECT	MECHANISM OF INTERACTION
Azole antifungals	Benzodiazepines, Oxidative Metabolism-class [alprazolam, chlordiazepoxide, clonazepam, clorazepate, diazepam,estazolam, flurazepam, halazepam, midazolam,quazepam, triazolam]	Increased concentrations of benzodiazepine. Prolonged CNS depression and psychomotor impairment.	Azole Antifungals inhibit CYP3A4 mediated benzodiazepine metabolism. Azole Antifungals decrease reanal excretion of some benzodiazepine
	buspirone	Increased effects of buspirone.	CYP3A4 inhibition by Azole
	cyclosporine	Increased concentrations of cyclosporine.	Inhibtion of CYP3A4 mediated cyclosporine metabolism by Azole Antifungals. Also inhibition of p-glycoprotein that interfere with cyclosporine transport
	dexamethasone	Increased effects of dexamethasone.	Inhibition of CYP3A4 by Azole Antifungals

DRUG	DRUG INTERACTION	EFFECT	MECHANISM OF INTERACTION
	haloperidol	Increased concentrations of haloperidol.	Inhibition of CYP3A4 mediated haloperidol metabolism by Azole
	HMG-CoA Reductase Inhibitors [fluvastatin, lovastatin, simvastatin]	Increased risk of rhabdomyolysis.	Azole Antifungals inhibit CYP2C9 and CYP3A4 mediated HMG-CoA Reductase Inhibitors metabolism
	hydrocortisone	Increased effects of hydrocortisone.	Inhibition of CYP3A4 by Azole Antifungals
	Rifamycins [rifabutin, rifampin, rifapentine]	Decreased concentrations of azole antifungal. Increase serum concentration of rifamycin	Induction of CYP3A4 by rifamycin. Inhibition of CYP isoenzymes by azole antifungal.
	Protease Inhibitors [indinavir, ritonavir, saquinavir]	Increase serum concentration of protease inhibitors.	Inhibition of CYP3A4 by azol Antifungals additionally for itraconazole and ketoconazole to inhibit p-glycoprotein
	Proton Pump Inhibitors[esome	Decrease serum concentration of	Decreased GI absorption of Azole

DRUG	DRUG INTERACTION	EFFECT	MECHANISM OF INTERACTION
	prazole, lansoprazole, omeprazole, pantoprazole, rabeprazole]	Azole antifungals. Increase serum concentration of Proton Pump Inhibitors	antifungals. Azole inhibit CYP3A4 mediated Proton Pump Inhibitors metabolism,
	sirolimus	Increased concentrations of sirolimus.	Inhibition of CYP3A4 mediated tacrolimus metabolism by Azole Antifungals
	Sulfonylureas [acetohexamide, chlorpropamide, glipizide, glyburide, tolazamide, tolbutamide]	Increased hypoglycemic effects of Sulfonylureas	Inhibition of CYP2C9 isoenzymes by azole antifungal
	tacrolimus	Increased concentrations of tacrolimus.	Inhibition of CYP3A4 mediated tacrolimus metabolism by Azole Antifungals
	quinidine	Increased concentrations of quinidine.	Inhibition of CYP3A4 mediated quinidine metabolism by azole derivatives
	warfarin	Increased effects of warfarin.	Inhibition of CYP3A4 mediated warfarin metabolism by

DRUG	DRUG INTERACTION	EFFECT	MECHANISM OF INTERACTION
			azole Azole Antifungals
Fluconazole *(See also* Azole Antifungals*)*	cisapride	Increase serum concentration of cisapride, hence, increase the risk of cardiac arrhythmias (eg. Torsades de pointes	Inhibition of CYP3A4 isoenzymes by fluconazole
	clopidogrel	Decrease the active metabolites of clopidogril, decrease platelet inhibition and increase the concentration of (parent) clopidogrel.	CYP2C19 inhibition by fluconazole
	Digoxin, digitoxin	Increase risk of digoxin toxicity, increase serum concentration of digoxin to 25%	Inhibition of p-glycoprotein by fluconazole
	Calcium channel blockers (amlodipine, diltiazem, isradipine, felodipine, nicardipine, nifedipine, verapamil)	Increase serum concentration of calcium channel blockers, enhance side effect like edema of leg and anklel	Inhibition of CYP3A4 by fluconazole

DRUG	DRUG INTERACTION	EFFECT	MECHANISM OF INTERACTION
DRUG	DRUG INTERACTION	EFFECT	MECHANISM OF INTERACTION
	Hydantoins [ethotoinfosphenytoin, mephenytoin, phenytoin]	Increased effects of hydantoin.	Inhibition of CYP2C9 by fluconazole
	thioridazine	Increase risk of ventricular fibrillation	Augmentation of QTc—prolongation by both drugs
	quinine	Increase risk of ventricular fibrillation	Augmentation of QTc—prolongation by both drugs

Itraconazole

DRUG	DRUG INTERACTION	EFFECT	MECHANISM OF INTERACTION
Itraconazole (See also Azole Antifungals)	cisapride	Increase serum concentration of cisapride, hence, increase the risk of cardiac arrhythmias (eg. Torsades de pointes	Inhibition of CYP3A4 isoenzymes by Itraconazole
	clopidogrel	Decrease the active metabolites of clopidogril,	CYP2C19 inhibition by Itraconazole

DRUG	DRUG INTERACTION	EFFECT	MECHANISM OF INTERACTION
		decrease platelet inhibition and increase the concentration of (parent) clopidogrel.	
	Calcium channel blockers(amlodipine, diltiazem, isradipine, felodipine, nicardipine, nifedipine, verapamil)	Increase serum concentration of calcium channel blockers, enhance side effect like edema of leg and anklel	Inhibition of CYP3A4 by Itraconazole
	Didanosine	Decreased GI absorption of itraconazole.	The buffer system of didanosine may reduce absorption of itraconazole by increasing gastric pH
	Digoxin	Increased concentrations of digoxin .	Itraconazole induce changes in urinary clearace of digoxin and inhibition of p-glycoprotein
	Hydantoins [ethotoinfosphenytoin, mephenytoin, phenytoin]	Increased effects of hydantoin.	Inhibition of CYP2C9 by itraconazole

Ketoconazole

DRUG	DRUG INTERACTION	EFFECT	MECHANISM OF INTERACTION
Ketoconazole *(See also* Azole Antifungals*)*	cisapride	Increase serum concentration of cisapride, hence, increase the risk of cardiac arrhythmias (eg. Torsades de pointes	Inhibition of CYP3A4 isoenzymes by ketoconazole
	clopidogrel	Decrease the active metabolites of clopidogril, decrease platelet inhibition and increase the concentration of (parent) clopidogrel.	CYP2C19 inhibition by ketoconazole
	Calcium channel blockers (amlodipine, diltiazem, isradipine, felodipine, nicardipine, nifedipine, verapamil)	Increase serum concentration of calcium channel blockers, enhance side effect like edema of leg and anklel	Inhibition of CYP3A4 by ketoconazole
	Didanosine	Decreased GI absorption of ketoconazole.	The buffer system of didanosine may reduce absorption of ketoconazole by increasing gastric pH.

DRUG	DRUG INTERACTION	EFFECT	MECHANISM OF INTERACTION
	Digoxin, digitoxin	Increase risk of digoxin toxicity, increase serum concentration of digoxin to 25%	Inhibition of p-glycoprotein by ketoconazole
	Histamine H2-Antagonists[cime tidine, famotidine, nizatidine, ranitidine]	Decreased GI absorptionof ketoconazole.	Ketoconazole required acidic media for dissolution, Histamine H2-Antagonists decrease the rate of absorption of Ketoconazole
	Hydantoins [ethotoinfosphen ytoin, mephenytoin, phenytoin]	Decreased effects of ketoconazole. Increase serum concentration of Hydantoins	Induction of CYP3A4 by Hydantoins that mediated metabolism of ketoconazole. Inhibition of CYP2C9 and or CYP2C19 mediated metabolism of Hydantoins by azole antifungal
	Antacids[aluminu m hydroxide, aluminum-magnesium hydroxide, magnesium hydroxide,	Decrease concentration of Ketoconazole	Ketoconazole tablets require an acidic media for dissolution, Antacids decrease Ketoconazole dissolution that decrease its

DRUG	DRUG INTERACTION	EFFECT	MECHANISM OF INTERACTION
	sodium bicarbonate]		absorption
Voriconazole (*See also* Azole Antifungals*)*	Barbiturates [amobarbital, aprobarbital, butabarbital, butalbital, mephobarbital, pentobarbital, phenobarbital, primidone, secobarbital]	Decreased concentrations of voriconazole. therapy failure	Induction of metablizing enzymes for Voriconazole by Barbiturate
	Ergot Alkaloids	Increased risk of ergot toxicity (peripheral ischemia, peripheral vasospasm).	Inhibition of CYP3A4 mediated ergot metabolism by Voriconazole

Griseofulvin

DRUG	DRUG INTERACTION	EFFECT	MECHANISM OF INTERACTION
Griseofulvin	alcohol	Disulferam like reaction	Griseofulvin inhibit aldehyde dehydrogenase thus inhibit alcohol metabolism
	Barbiturates [amobarbital,	Decreased concentrationsof	Decrease absorption of

DRUG	DRUG INTERACTION	EFFECT	MECHANISM OF INTERACTION
	aprobarbital, butabarbital, butalbital, mephobarbital, pentobarbital, phenobarbital, primidone, secobarbital]	griseofulvin	griseofulvin
	Salicylates (aminosalisylate, aspirin, salsalate, sodium salisylate	Decrease therapeutic effects of salisylate	Decrease absorption of salisylate
	Contraceptive (progesterons)	Contraceptive failure is possible	Induction of CYP metabolism of progesterone (probably estrogen)
	Warfarin	Decreased effects of warfarin.	Induction of CYP3A4 and CYP2C9 by griseofulvin

CARDIOVASCULAR AGENTS

ANTIHYPERTENSIVE DRUGS

Adrenergic drugs

Clonidine

DRUG	DRUG INTERACTION	EFFECT	MECHANISM OF INTERACTION
Clonidine	Amphetamines	Decrease the antihypertensive effect of clonidine	Amphetamines known to cause modest increase in average blood pressure and heart rate
	Beta-Blockers [acebutolol, atenolol, betaxolol, carteolol, esmolol, metoprolol, nadolol, penbutolol, pindolol, propranolol, timolol]	Enhance the rebound hypertension if clonidine is abruptly withdrawn	Increase circulating catecholamines (centrally suppressed by clonidine), Beta-Blockers unopposed the vasoconstrictor of catecholamines
	Tricyclic Antidepressants [amitriptyline, amoxapine, clomipramine, desipramine, doxepin, imipramine, nortriptyline, protriptyline,	Loss of blood pressure control. Increased risk of hypertensive crisis.	The ability of tricyclic antidepressants to enhance the pressor response to catecholamines

DRUG	DRUG INTERACTION	EFFECT	MECHANISM OF INTERACTION
	trimipramine]		

Methyldopa

DRUG	DRUG INTERACTION	EFFECT	MECHANISM OF INTERACTION
Methyldopa	MAO inhibitors[isocarb oxazid, phenelzine, selegiline, tranylcypromine]	Enhance adverse/toxic effect of methyldopa	involve excessive sympathetic stimulation in the central nervous system.
	Iron Salts (Oral) [ferrous fumarate, ferrous sulfate, iron polysaccharide]	Decrease therapeutic effect of methyldopa	Formation of poorly absorbed complex
	lithium	Increase toxic effect of lithium without change in serum concentration of lithium	Unknown
	Sympathomimeti cs[dobutamine, dopamine, Discontinueephe drine, epinephrine, mephentermine,	Increased blood pressure.	Unknown

DRUG	DRUG INTERACTION	EFFECT	MECHANISM OF INTERACTION
	metaraminol, methoxamine, norepinephrine, phenylephrine, pseudoephedrine]		

Alpha 1-blockers

DRUG	DRUG INTERACTION	EFFECT	MECHANISM OF INTERACTION
Alpha 1-blockers (Prazosin, doxazocin, phenoxybenzamine, phyntolamine, tamsulosin, terazosin)	Phosphodiesterase inhibitors (sildenafil, tadalafil, vardenafil)	Enhance the hypotensive effect of prazosin	Additive vasodilating effect
	Beta-Blockers [acebutolol, atenolol, betaxolol, bisoprolol, carteolol, esmolol, metoprolol, nadolol, penbutolol, pindolol, propranolol,	Increased postural hypotension.	Additive postural hypotension effect of both drugs

DRUG	DRUG INTERACTION	EFFECT	MECHANISM OF INTERACTION
	sotalol, timolol]		
	Verapamil	Enhance the hypotensive effect of Verapamil	Increase serum concentration of Alpha 1-blockers. Verapamil decrease metabolism of Alpha 1-blockers

Angiotensin Converting Enzyme Inhibitors (ACEIs

Benazepril, Captopril, Enalapril, Fosinopril, Lisinopril, Moexipril, Perindopril, Quinapril, Trandolapril

DRUG	DRUG INTERACTION	EFFECT	MECHANISM OF INTERACTION
Angiotensin Converting Enzyme Inhibitor ACE Inhibitors	allopurinol	Enhance the potential for allergic or hypersensitivity reactions to allopuranol (stevens-johnson syndrome)	unknown but impaired renal function may be a predisposing factor
	azathioprine	Enhance the neutropenic effect of Azathioprine	Related to the additive toxic effect of individual agents on bone marrow
	antacid	Decrease serum concentration of ACEI	Decrease absorption of ACEI
	cyclosporine	Increase risk of	Cyclosporine cause

DRUG	DRUG INTERACTION	EFFECT	MECHANISM OF INTERACTION
		cyclosporine nephrotoxicity	renal afferent vessel constriction, increasing the kidney reliance on angiotensin II to maintain adequate perfusion. ACEI decrease angiotensin II concentration
	Iron-dextran complex	Increase adverse/ toxic effect of iron dextran complex. Increase risk of anaphylactic-type reactions	unknown
	NSAIDs [diclofenac, ibuprofen, indomethacin, ketorolac, meloxicam, naproxen, piroxicam, sulindac]	Decreased effects of angiotensin converting enzyme inhibitor.	Effect on vascular tone and fluid homeostasis
	insulin	Enhance hypoglycemic effect of insulin	ACEI have various effect both islet structure and function as well as enhancing insulin sensitivity
	Lithium	Increased concentrations/tox icity of lithium.	unknown

DRUG	DRUG INTERACTION	EFFECT	MECHANISM OF INTERACTION
	Potassium-Sparing Diuretics	Elevated serum potassium.	Additive hyperkalemic effect of both drugs
	sulfonylureas	Enhance hypoglycemic effect of sulphonylureas	ACEI have various effect both islet structure and function as well ason the physiologic response to hypoglycemia
	trimethoprim	Enhance the hyperkalemic effect of ACEI	Both drug reduce renal potassium excretion

Angiotensin IIReceptor Blockers(ARBs)

Candesartan, Eprosartan, Irbesartan, Losartan, Olmesartan, Telmisartan, Valsartan

DRUG	DRUG INTERACTION	EFFECT	MECHANISM OF INTERACTION
Angiotensin IIReceptor Blockers	Lithium	Increased concentrationsof lithium.	Decrease renal elimination of Lithium
	trimethoprim	Enhance the hyperkalemic effect of Angiotensin IIReceptor Blockers	Both drug reduce renal potassium excretion

Beta-Blockers:

Cardio-Selective [Acebutolol, Atenolol, Betaxolol, Bisoprolol, Esmolol, Metoprolol, Nadolol];

Noncardio-Selective [Carteolol, Carvedilol, Labetalol, Penbutolol, Pindolol, Propranolol, Sotalol, Timolol]

Cardio-Selective and Noncardio-Selective Beta-Blockers-class

DRUG	DRUG INTERACTION	EFFECT	MECHANISM OF INTERACTION
Cardio-Selective and Noncardio-Selective Beta-Blockers-class	Alpha 1-blockers (Prazosin, doxazocin, phenoxybenzamine, phyntolamine, tamsulosin, terazosin)	Increased postural hypotension.	Additive postural hypotension effect of both drugs
	antacid	Decrease serum concentration of B—blockers except for metoprolol	delayed gastric emptying time by antacid or the formation of complex
	Barbiturates [amobarbital, aprobarbital, butabarbital, butalbital, mephobarbital, pentobarbital, phenobarbital, primidone, secobarbital]	Decreased bioavailability of beta-blocker.	Induction of metabolism that is not excreted unchanged in urine
	Cimetidine	Increased	inhibition of

DRUG	DRUG INTERACTION	EFFECT	MECHANISM OF INTERACTION
		concentrations of beta-blocker.	metabolism that is not excreted unchanged in urine
	Clonidine	Enhance the rebound hypertension if clonidine is abruptly withdrawn	Increase circulating catecholamines (centrally suppressed by clonidine), Beta-Blockers unopposed the vasoconstrictor of catecholamines
	Hydralazine	Increased concentrations of both drugs (metoprolol, propranolol).	reduced hepatic blood flow resulting in decreased biotransformation of beta blockers that undergo extensive first-pass metabolism
	Propafenone	Increased effects of beta-blocker (metoprolol, propanolol).	Propafenone possesses beta-blocking activity. Propafenone decrease the CYP2D6 metabolism of beta-blocker
	Quinidine	Increased effects of beta-blocker (atenolol, propranolol, betametoprolol,	Quinidine inhibit CYP2D6 mediated metabolism of beta-blocker

DRUG	DRUG INTERACTION	EFFECT	MECHANISM OF INTERACTION
		timolol).	
	Rifamycins	Decreased effects of beta-blocker (atenolol, bisoprolol, metoprolol, propranolol).	Induction of CYP3A4 isoenzyme by Rifamycins
	Verapamil	Increased effects of both drugs.(bradycardia, signs of heart failure	Both have negative inotropic action on 5the heart

Noncardio-Selective Beta-Blockers-class

DRUG	DRUG INTERACTION	EFFECT	MECHANISM OF INTERACTION
Noncardio-Selective Beta-Blockers-class	antacid	Decrease serum concentration of B—blockers	delayed gastric emptying time by antacid or the formation of complex
	Epinephrine	Initial hypertensive episode, followed by reflex bradycardia.	Non selective beta blockers unopposed alpha effects and result in vasoconstriction, a subsequent decrease in heart rate occurs due to increased vagal

DRUG	DRUG INTERACTION	EFFECT	MECHANISM OF INTERACTION
			tone(reflex)
	Ergot	Increased risk of ergot toxicity (peripheral ischemia, gangrene).	unknown, but may involve blockade of beta-2-mediated (i.e., sympathetic) vasodilatation. In addition, beta-1 blockade reduces cardiac output, which can diminish blood flow and exacerbate ergot-induced vasospasm. Peripheral ischemia, hypertension with chest pain, gangrene resulting in surgical amputation, and migraine exacerbation have been described in suspected cases of the interaction.
	Insulin	Prolonged hypoglycemia with masking of hypoglycemic signs/symptoms (tachycardia)	Blocking of beta receptors in pancrease that regulate insulin release, and inhibition of tackycardia mediated by Epinephrine
	NSAIDs [diclofenac,	Decreased antihypertensive	Effect on vascular tone and fluid

DRUG	DRUG INTERACTION	EFFECT	MECHANISM OF INTERACTION
	etodolac, fenoprofen, flurbiprofen, ibuprofen, indomethacin, ketoprofen, ketorolac, meclofenamate, nabumetone, naproxen, oxaprozin, piroxicam, sulindac, tolmetin]	effects of beta-blocker.	homeostasis
	Prazosin	Increased postural hypotension.	Additive postural hypotension effect of both drugs
	Theophylline	Increased concentrations of theophylline. Pharmacologic antagonism may decrease effects of one or both drugs.	Decrease theophylline clearance, inhibition of CYP1A2 and or 3A4 by propranolol mediated theophylline metabolism and antagonism of theophylline effect by beta receptor blocking

DRUG	DRUG INTERACTION	EFFECT	MECHANISM OF INTERACTION
Atenolol *(See also Cardio-Selective and Noncardio-Selective Beta-Blockers-class)*	Ampicillin	Decreased effects of atenolol.	due to impaired gastrointestinal absorption in the presence of ampicillin.
Carvedilol *(See also Cardio-Selective and Noncardio-Selective Beta-Blockers-class)*	Cyclosporine	Increased concentrations of cyclosporine.	Carvedolol mediated inhibition of p-glycoprotein that effect transport of cyclosporine
Labetalol *(See also Cardio-Selective and Noncardio-Selective Beta-Blockers-class)*	Inhalation Anesthetics [desflurane, enflurane, halothane, isoflurane, sevoflurane]	Excessive hypotension.	The antihypertensive effects of inhalational anesthetics and some beta-blockers may be additive.
Metoprolol *(See also Cardio-Selective and Noncardio-Selective Beta-Blockers-class)*	Lidocaine	Increased effects of Lidocaine.	Metoprolol decrease cardiac output and thus reducing hepatic blood flow and decrease the presentation of lidocaine to the hepatocytes that decrase its

DRUG	DRUG INTERACTION	EFFECT	MECHANISM OF INTERACTION
			metabolism
	Thioamines [methimazole, propylthiouracil]	Increased effects of metoprolol.	The clearance of some beta-blockers with high extraction ratios may be reduced when a euthyroid state is achieved after the addition of antithyroid agents.
Nadolol *(See also Cardio-Selective and Noncardio-Selective Beta-Blockers-class)*	Lidocaine	Increased concentrations of lidocaine.	Metoprolol decrease cardiac output and thus reducing hepatic blood flow and decrease the presentation of lidocaine to the hepatocytes that decrase its metabolism
Pindolol *(See also Cardio-Selective and Noncardio-Selective Beta-Blockers-class)*	Lidocaine	ncreased concentrations of lidocaine.	Metoprolol decrease cardiac output and thus reducing hepatic blood flow and decrease the presentation of lidocaine to the hepatocytes that decrase its metabolism
	Phenothiazines [chlorpromazine, thioridazine]	Increased effects of one or both drugs.	Each drug inhibit the metabolism of other.

DRUG	DRUG INTERACTION	EFFECT	MECHANISM OF INTERACTION
			Both drug produce hypotension and thus hypotension is augmented
Propranolol *(See also Cardio-Selective and Noncardio-Selective Beta-Blockers-class)*	Lidocaine	ncreased concentrations of lidocaine.	Metoprolol decrease cardiac output and thus reducing hepatic blood flow and decrease the presentation of lidocaine to the hepatocytes that decrase its metabolism
	Phenothiazines [chlorpromazine, thioridazine]	Increased effects of one or both drugs.	Each drug inhibit the metabolism of other. Both drug produce hypotension and thus hypotension is augmented
	Thioamines [methimazole, propylthiouracil]	Increased effects of propranolol.	The clearance of some beta-blockers with high extraction ratios may be reduced when a euthyroid state is achieved after the addition of antithyroid agents.
	zileuton	Increase effect of	Increase B—

DRUG	DRUG INTERACTION	EFFECT	MECHANISM OF INTERACTION
		propranolol	blockage accompanied by concomitant use of these drugs
Sotalol(See also Cardio-Selective and Noncardio-Selective Beta-Blockers-class)	Quinolones [gatifloxacin, moxifloxacin, sparfloxacin]	Increased risk of cardiac arrhythmias, including torsades de pointes.	Enhance the QTc-prolongatoion for each drug.

Calcium-Channel Blockers (CCBs):

Amlodipine, Diltiazem, Felodipine, Isradipine, Nicardipine, Nifedipine, Nimodipine, Nisoldipine, Verapamil

Diltiazem

DRUG	DRUG INTERACTION	EFFECT	MECHANISM OF INTERACTION
Calcium channel blockers (amlodipine, diltiazem, isradipine, felodipine, nicardipine, nifedipine, verapamil)	Azole Antifungals: Fluconazole, Itraconazole, Ketoconazole, Miconazole, Voriconazole	Increase serum concentration of calcium channel blockers, enhance side effect like edema of leg and anklel	Inhibition of CYP3A4 by Azole Antifungals
	Barbiturates [amobarbital, aprobarbital, butabarbital, butalbital,	Decrease effect of Calcium channel blockers	induction of CYP3A4 isoenzyme by barbiturates

DRUG	DRUG INTERACTION	EFFECT	MECHANISM OF INTERACTION
	mephobarbital, pentobarbital, phenobarbital, primidone, secobarbital]		
	cimetidine	Increase bioavailability of Calcium channel blockers	Inhibition of CYP3A4 by cimetidine
	carbamazepine	Increased concentrations of carbamazepine. Decrease concentration of Calcium channel blockers	Inhibition of CYP isoenzymes mediated carbamazepine metabolism by Calcium channel blockers. Induction of CYP isoenzymes mediated Calcium channel blockers metabolism
	Cyclosporine	Increased concentrations of Calcium channel blockers.	Inhibition of CYP3A4 by Cyclosporine decrease Calcium channel blockers metabolism
	Macrolide antibiotics(clarith romycine, erythomycine, telithromycine)	increase serum concentration of calcium channel blocker, increase risk of	Inhibition of CYP3A4 by macrolides

DRUG	DRUG INTERACTION	EFFECT	MECHANISM OF INTERACTION
	Exceptions: azithromycin, spiromycim	fatigue, dizziness, bradycardia, hypotension	
	phenytoin	Increase phenytoin toxicity	calcium channel blockers may effect phenytoin clearance, either by CYP3A4 inhibition or by change in hepatic blood flow
	Rifamycins [rifabutin, rifampin]	Decrease therapeutic effect of Calcium channel blockers	Induction of CYP3A4 isoenzymes, especially in the intestinal mucosa.(inhibit metabolism and absorption)
Diltiazem *(See also* Calcium channel blockers*)*	Benzodiazepines	Increased effects of benzodiazepine (diazepam, midazolam, triazolam). Prolonged sedation and respiratory depression.	Inhibition of CYP3A4 by diltiazem
	cyclosporine	Increased concentrations of Calcium channel blockers.	Inhibition of CYP3A4 by Cyclosporine decrease Calcium channel blockers

DRUG	DRUG INTERACTION	EFFECT	MECHANISM OF INTERACTION
			metabolism
	HMG-CoA Reductase Inhibitors	Increased risk of rhabdomyolysis. [Exceptions: fluvastatin, pravastatin]	Inhibition of CYP3A4-mediated HMG-CoA Reductase Inhibitors metabolism by diltiazem
	Quinidine	Increased concentrations of quinidine (increased QTc, PR interval, decrease heart rate/ blood pressure).	Inhibition of CYP3A4 mediated Quinidine metabolism by diltiazem
	Sirolimus	Increased concentrations of sirolimus.	Inhibition of CYP3A4 by diltiazem
	Tacrolimus	Increased concentrations of tacrolimus.	Inhibition of CYP3A4 by diltiazem
	Theophyllines[am inophylline, oxtriphylline, theophylline]	Increased concentrationsof theophylline.	Inhibition of CYP3A4 by diltiazem

Felodipine

DRUG	DRUG INTERACTION	EFFECT	MECHANISM OF INTERACTION
Felodipine *(See also* Calcium channel blockers*)*	Hydantoins [ethotoin, fosphenytoin, mephenytoin, phenytoin]	Increase phenytoin toxicity	calcium channel blockers may effect phenytoin clearance, either by CYP3A4 inhibition or by change in hepatic blood flow

Nicardipine

DRUG	DRUG INTERACTION	EFFECT	MECHANISM OF INTERACTION
Nicardipine *(See also* Calcium channel blockers*)*	Cyclosporine	Increased concentrations of Calcium channel blockers.	Inhibition of CYP3A4 by Cyclosporine decrease Calcium channel blockers metabolism
Nifedipine *(See also* Calcium channel blockers*)*	Cimetidine	Increase bioavailability of Calcium channel blockers	Inhibition of CYP3A4 by cimetidine
	Tacrolimus	Increased concentrations of tacrolimus.	Inhibition of CYP3A4 by Nifedipine
Nisoldipine	Hydantoins	Increase phenytoin	calcium channel

DRUG	DRUG INTERACTION	EFFECT	MECHANISM OF INTERACTION
(See also Calcium channel blockers)	[ethotoin, fosphenytoin, mephenytoin, phenytoin]	toxicity	blockers may effect phenytoin clearance, either by CYP3A4 inhibition or by change in hepatic blood flow

Verapamil

DRUG	DRUG INTERACTION	EFFECT	MECHANISM OF INTERACTION
Verapamil (See also Calcium channel blockers)	Beta-Blockers	Increased effects of both drugs.(bradycardia, signs of heart failure	Both have negative inotropic action on 5the heart
	Calcium Salts[calcium acetate, calcium carbonate, calcium chloride, calcium citrate, calcium glubionate, calcium gluconate, calcium glycerophosphate, calcium lactate, calcium levulinate, tricalcium phosphate]	Reverse clinical effects and toxicities of verapamil.	Calcium-containing products may decrease the effectiveness of calcium channel blockers by saturating calcium channels with calcium.

DRUG	DRUG INTERACTION	EFFECT	MECHANISM OF INTERACTION
	carbamazepine	Increased concentrations of carbamazepine. Decrease concentration of Verapamil	Inhibition of CYP isoenzymes mediated carbamazepine metabolism by Verapamil. Induction of CYP isoenzymes mediated Verapamil metabolism
	Cyclosporine	Increased concentrations of Calcium channel blockers.	Inhibition of CYP3A4 by Cyclosporine decrease Calcium channel blockers metabolism
	Digoxin	Increase serum concentration of digoxin. Enhance the AV—blocking effect of cardiac glycosides by Calcium channel blockers	Decrease in cardiac glycosides clearance by Calcium channel blockers
	Ethanol	Increase therapeutic/toxic effect of verapamil	Inhibition of CYP3A4 by Ethanol
	HMG-CoA Reductase Inhibitors	Increased risk of rhabdomyolysis. [Exceptions:	Inhibition of CYP3A4-mediated HMG-CoA

DRUG	DRUG INTERACTION	EFFECT	MECHANISM OF INTERACTION
		fluvastatin, pravastatin]	Reductase Inhibitors metabolism by verapamil
	atracurium, doxacurium, mivacurium pancuronium, pipecuronium, tubocurarine, vecuronium	Increased nondepolarizing muscle relaxant effects (prolonged respiratory depression).	Calcium channel blockers decrease the release of acetylcholine by reducing the concentration of calcium within nerve endings
	Alpha 1-blockers (Prazosin, doxazocin, phenoxybenzami ne, phyntolamine, tamsulosin, terazosin)	Enhance the hypotensive effect of Verapamil	Increase serum concentration of Alpha 1-blockers. Verapamil decrease metabolism of Alpha 1-blockers
	Quinidine	Increased concentrations of quinidine Increased risk of cardiac arrhythimas and hypotension.	Inhibition of CYP3A4 mediated Quinidine metabolism by Verapamil

Antiarrhythmic Agents

Amiodarone

DRUG	DRUG INTERACTION	EFFECT	MECHANISM OF INTERACTION
Amiodarone	Cholestyramine	Decrease effect of amiodarone	Binding of amiodarone and Cholestyramine in GIT that inhibit its absorption
	Cyclosporine	Increased concentrations/toxicity of cyclosporine.	Inhibition of cyclosporine metabolism
	Digoxin	Increased concentrations/toxicity of digoxin.	Amiodarone decrease digoxin clearance by renal and non renal as well as amiodarone associated hypothyroidism has been suggested to effect digoxin clearance
	Fentanyl	Increase concentration of Fentanyl.Increased risk of profound bradycardia, sinus arrest, and hypotension.	Inhibition of CYP3A4 mediated Fentanyl metabolism by amiodarone
	HMG-CoA Reductase Inhibitors	Enhance risk of severe myopathy and	Amiodarone decrease metabolism of

DRUG	DRUG INTERACTION	EFFECT	MECHANISM OF INTERACTION
	[fluvastatin, lovastatin, simvastatin]	rhabdomyolysis	HMG-CoA Reductase Inhibitors by by CYP3A4 inhibition
	Hydantoins [ethotoin, fosphenytoin, mephenytoin, phenytoin]	Increased concentrations of hydantoin. Decreased concentrations of amiodarone.	Inhibition of CYP2C9 mediated hydantoin metabolism by amiodarone. CYP isenzyme induction by Hydantoins
	loratadine	Increase serum concentration of loratadine, enhance risk of QT interval prolongation and torsades de pointes	Inhibition of CYP3A4 by amiodarone
	Procainamide	Increased concentrations of procainamide and N-acetylprocainamide. Enhance QTc prolongation	Inhibition of CYP3A4 by amiodarone
	Protease Inhibitors[indinavir, ritonavir]	Increased concentrations of amiodarone.	Potent inhibitionn of CYP3A4 by Protease Inhibitors
	Quinidine	Increased concentrations of	Inhibition of CYP3A4 and

DRUG	DRUG INTERACTION	EFFECT	MECHANISM OF INTERACTION
		quinidine. Increased risk of cardiac arrhythimas.	possibly CYP2D6 by amiodarone
	Quinolones [gatifloxacin, moxifloxacin, sparfloxacin]	Increased risk of cardiac arrhythmias, including torsades de pointes.	Enhance the QTc-prolongatoion for each drug
	thioridazine	Enhance QTc—prolongation effect of amiodarone	Thioridazine and amiodarone both cause prolongation of QTc—interval
	Theophylline class	Increase toxic effect of theophylline	Inhibition of enzymes responsible for theophylline metabolism
	Warfarin	Increased the anticoagulant effects of warfarin.	Inhibition of CYP isoenzymes by amiodarone, and the iodine content of amiodarone may cause hyperthyroidism following chronic use may increase body sensitivity to warfarin

Disopyramide

DRUG	DRUG INTERACTION	EFFECT	MECHANISM OF INTERACTION
Disopyramide	Hydantoins [ethotoin, fosphenytoin, mephenytoin, phenytoin]	Decreased concentrationsof disopyramide. Increased risk of anticholinergic effects.	CYP3A4 induction by Hydantoins
	Quinolones [gatifloxacin, moxifloxacin, sparfloxacin]	Increased risk of cardiac rrhythmias, including torsades de pointes.	Enhance the QTc-prolongatoion for each drug.
	Rifampin	Decreased concentrations of disopyramide.	CYP3A4 induction by rifampin

Flecainide

DRUG	DRUG INTERACTION	EFFECT	MECHANISM OF INTERACTION
Flecainide	Protease Inhibitors [indinavir, ritonavir]	Increased concentrations of flecainide.	Potent inhibitionn of CYP3A4 by Protease Inhibitors

Lidocaine

DRUG	DRUG INTERACTION	EFFECT	MECHANISM OF INTERACTION
Lidocaine	Beta-Blockers [atenolol, metoprolol, nadolol pindolol, propranolol]	Increased effects of Lidocaine.	Metoprolol decrease cardiac output and thus reducing hepatic blood flow and decrease the presentation of lidocaine to the hepatocytes that decrase its metabolism
	Cimetidine	Increased concentrations of lidocaine.	inhibition of hepatic CYP450 metabolism and reduced hepatic blood flow
	tamoxifen	Increase serum concentration of tamoxifen, decrease the formation of highly potent active metabolite of tamoxifen	Inhibition of CYP2D6 by lidocaine
	thioridazine	Increase serum concentration of thioridazine and enhance QTc intervals	Inhibition of CYP2D6 by lidocaine

Mexiletine

DRUG	DRUG INTERACTION	EFFECT	MECHANISM OF INTERACTION
Mexiletine	Hydantoins [ethotoin, fosphenytoin, mephenytoin, phenytoin]	Decreased concentrationsof mexiletine.	CYP3A4 induction by Hydantoins
	Theophylline	Increased concentrations of theophylline	Mexiletine inhibit CYP1A2, the primary metabolizing isoenzyme for theophylline

Procainamide

DRUG	DRUG INTERACTION	EFFECT	MECHANISM OF INTERACTION
Procainamide	Amiodarone	Increased concentrations of procainamide and N-acetylprocainamide. Enhance QTc prolongation	Inhibition of CYP3A4 by amiodarone
	Cimetidine	Increased concentrationsof procainamide and N-acetylprocainamide	Cimetidine decrease renal excretion of procainamide
	Ofloxacin	Increased	Competition for

DRUG	DRUG INTERACTION	EFFECT	MECHANISM OF INTERACTION
		concentrations of procainamide.	the excretion site in the kidney
	Quinolones [gatifloxacin, moxifloxacin, sparfloxacin]	Increased risk of cardiac arrhythmias, including torsades de pointes.	Enhance the QTc-prolongatoion for each drug.
	Trimethoprim	Increased concentrations of procainamide and N-acetylprocainamide.	Competition for the excretion site in the renal tubules

Propafenone

DRUG	DRUG INTERACTION	EFFECT	MECHANISM OF INTERACTION
Propafenone	Quinidine	Increased concentrations/ toxic effect of propafenone.	quinidine inhibit the CYP450 2D6-mediated metabolism of propafenone
	beta-blocker (metoprolol, propanolol)	Increased effects of beta-blocker (metoprolol, propanolol).	Propafenone possesses beta-blocking activity. Propafenone decrease the CYP2D6 metabolism of beta-blocker
	digoxin	Increased	inhibition of p-

DRUG	DRUG INTERACTION	EFFECT	MECHANISM OF INTERACTION
		concentrations/ toxic effect of digoxin.	glycoprotein that reducing glycoside transport

Quinidine

DRUG	DRUG INTERACTION	EFFECT	MECHANISM OF INTERACTION
Quinidine	Amiloride	Increased risk of cardiac rrhythmias and reversal of quinidine effects.	synergistic increase in sodium channel blockage.
	Amiodarone	Increased concentrations of quinidine. Increased risk of cardiac arrhythimas.	Inhibition of CYP3A4 and possibly CYP2D6 by amiodarone
	beta-blockers(atenolol, propranolol, betametoprolol, timolol).	Increased effects of beta-blocker (atenolol, propranolol, betametoprolol, timolol).	Quinidine inhibit CYP2D6 mediated metabolism of beta-blocker
	Barbiturates [amobarbital, aprobarbital, butabarbital, butalbital, mephobarbital, pentobarbital,	Decreased concentrations of quinidine and increase toxic effect (hepatotoxicity) of quinidine	Induction of CYP3A4 and CYP2C9 by barbiturates. Both barbiturates and Quinidine can

DRUG	DRUG INTERACTION	EFFECT	MECHANISM OF INTERACTION
	phenobarbital, primidone, secobarbital]		induce hepatotoxicity
	Cimetidin	Increasedconcentrations of quinidine.	Inhibition of CYP3A4 mediated Quinidine metabolism by quinidine
	Codeine	Decreased effects of codeine.	Inhibition of CYP2D6 mediated codeine metabolism by quinidine
	Digoxin	Increased concentrations of digoxin.	Displacement of digoxin from tissue binding site also inhibition of p-glycoprotein that reducing glycoside transport
	Diltiazem	Increased concentrations of quinidine (increased QTc, PR interval, decrease heart rate/ blood pressure).	Inhibition of CYP3A4 mediated Quinidine metabolism by Diltiazem
	Hydantoins [fosphenytoin, phenytoin]	Decreased concentrations/ therapeutic effect of quinidine.	Induction of CYP3A4 and CYP2C9 by Hydantoins
	Azole	Increased	Inhibition of

DRUG	DRUG INTERACTION	EFFECT	MECHANISM OF INTERACTION
	Antifungals:, Itraconazole, Miconazole, Voriconazole	concentrations/ toxic effect of quinidine.	CYP3A4 mediated quinidine metabolism by azole derivatives
	Antacids[aluminum hydroxide, aluminum- magnesium hydroxide, magnesium hydroxide, sodium bicarbonate]	Increased concentrations/ toxic effect of of quinidine.	Quinidine renal excretion decreased in alkaline urine produced by antacids
	Propafenone	Increased concentrations/ toxic effect of propafenone.	quinidine inhibit the CYP450 2D6- mediated metabolism of propafenone
	Quinolones [gatifloxacin, moxifloxacin, sparfloxacin]	Increased risk of cardiac arrhythmias, including torsades de pointes.	Enhance the QTc- prolongatoion for each drug.
	Rifamycins [rifabutin, rifampin]	Decreased concentrations/ effect of quinidine.	Induction of CYP3A4. Protein displacement of quinidine and increase clearance and metabolism quinidine
	Protease	Increased	Potent CYP3A4

DRUG	DRUG INTERACTION	EFFECT	MECHANISM OF INTERACTION
	Inhibitors [indinavir, ritonavir, saquinavir]	concentrations/ toxic effect of quinidine (life-threatening adverse effect).	inhibitors of protease inhibitors decrease metabolism of quinidine
	sucralfate	Decreased GI absorption of quinidine	Binding of both drug in the GIT and thereby decrease absorption of quinidine
	Verapamil	Increased concentrations of quinidine. Increased risk of cardiac arrhythimas and hypotension.	Inhibition of CYP3A4 mediated Quinidine metabolism by Verapamil
	Warfarin	Enhance the anticoagulant effects of warfarin.	unknown

Nitrates: Amyl Nitrite, Isosorbide Dinitrate, Isosorbide Mononitrate, Nitroglycerin

DRUG	DRUG INTERACTION	EFFECT	MECHANISM OF INTERACTION
Nitrates	Ergot	Increased standing systolic blood pressure. Pharmacologic antagonism between	Pharmacologic antagonism between dihydroergotamine and

DRUG	DRUG INTERACTION	EFFECT	MECHANISM OF INTERACTION
		dihydroergotamine and nitroglycerin may decrease antianginal effects of Nitrates.	Nitrates
	Phosphodiesterase-5Enzyme Inhibitors [sildenafil, tradalafil, vardenafil]	Severe hypotension.	Potentiation of the vasodilatory effect of cGMP.
Nitroglycerin (See also Nitrates)	Alteplase (tPA)	Decreased effects of tPA.	Nitroglycerin increase hepatic blood flow and increase clearance of alteplase
	heparin	Decrease serum concentration of heparin. Diminish the anticoagulant effect of heparin	Alteration of antithrombin III function and chang in heparin concentration by nitroglycerin

Digoxin

DRUG	DRUG INTERACTION	EFFECT	MECHANISM OF INTERACTION
Digoxin	Aminoglycosides [kanamycin, neomycin, paromomycin]	Decreased concentrations of digoxin.	Only with oral aminoglycosides that decrease absorption of digoxin
	Aminoquinolines (antimalarial)(chl oroquine, hydroxychloroqui ne, primaquine	Increase serum/toxic effect of digoxin	Inhibition of p-glycoprotein by Aminoquinolines thus less digoxin available for metabolism
	Amiodarone	Increased concentrations/tox icity of digoxin.	Amiodarone decrease digoxin clearance by renal and non renal as well as amiodarone associated hypothyroidism has been suggested to effect digoxin clearance
	Antineoplastic Agents[bleomyci n, carmustine, cyclophosphamid e, cytarabine, doxorubicin, methotrexate, vincristine]	Decreased concentrations of digoxin.	1.Interference with digoxin tablet dissolution. 2.also possible that intestinal epithelial toxicity plays arole 3. increase hepatic p-glycoprotein

DRUG	DRUG INTERACTION	EFFECT	MECHANISM OF INTERACTION
	Bepridil	Increased concentrations of digoxin. Increased negative chronotropic effects.	Calcium channel blockers induce decrease in cardiac glycosides clearance
	Cholestyramine	Decreased concentrations of digoxin.	Cholestyramine bind digoxin in the GI tract, that inhibit digoxin absorption
	Cyclosporine	Increased concentrations of digoxin.	Cyclosporine inhibit p-glycoprotein activity that decrease the presentation of digoxin to the metabolic enzymes
	fluconazole	Increase risk of digoxin toxicity, increase serum concentration of digoxin to 25%	Inhibition of p-glycoprotein by fluconazole
	Indomethacin	Increased concentrations of digoxin in premature infants.	Decrease in renal perfusion resultfrom inhibition of prostaglandin decrease digoxin clearance
	Itraconazole	Increase risk of digoxin toxicity, increase serum	Inhibition of p-glycoprotein by Itraconazole and

DRUG	DRUG INTERACTION	EFFECT	MECHANISM OF INTERACTION
		concentration of digoxin to 25%	induce changes in urinay clearance of digoxin
	Loop Diuretics [bumetanide, ethacrynic acid, furosemide]	Increased risk of arrhythmias.	Hypokalemia and possibly hypomagnesemia cased by Loop Diuretics
	Macrolide Antibiotics [clarithromycin, erythromycin]	Increased concentrations/ toxic effect of digoxin.	Macrolide Antibiotics inhibit intestina and renal p-glycoprotein. Also macrolide might eradicate normal flora (ie.Eubacterium Lentum) that degrade some digoxin prior absorption, thus leaving greater quantity to be absorbed
	Metoclopramide	Decreased concentrations of digoxin.	metoclopramide-induced stimulation of gastric motility, which may decrease digoxin absorption. Rapidly dissolving preparations such as digoxin solution in capsules do not appear to be affected.

DRUG	DRUG INTERACTION	EFFECT	MECHANISM OF INTERACTION
	Penicillamine	Decreased concentrations of digoxin.	unknown
	Propafenone	Increased concentrations/ toxic effect of digoxin.	inhibition of p-glycoprotein that reducing glycoside transport
	Quinidine	Increased concentrations/ toxic effect of digoxin.	Displacement of digoxin from tissue binding site also inhibition of p-glycoprotein that reducing glycoside transport
	Quinine	Increased concentrations/ toxic effect of digoxin.	Quinine reduce clearance (ninrenal) of digoxin
	Spironolactone	Decreased inotropic effects of digoxin.	spironolactone may have a negative inotropic side effect.
	sucralfate	Decrease effect of digoxin	Binding of both drug in the GIT and thereby decrease absorption of digoxin
	Tetracyclines [demeclocycline, doxycycline,	Increased concentrations/ toxic effect of	tetracyclines reduces gut flora that would

DRUG	DRUG INTERACTION	EFFECT	MECHANISM OF INTERACTION
	minocycline, oxytetracycline, tetracycline]	digoxin.	metabolize some digoxin prior the absorption
	Thiazide Diuretics [bendroflumethiazide, chlorothiazide, chlorthalidone, hydrochlorothiazide, hydroflumethiazid, indapamide, methyclothiazide, metolazone, polythiazide, trichlormethiazide]	Increased risk of arrhythmias.	Hypokalemia and possibly hypomagnesemia cased by Thiazide Diuretics
	Thioamines [methimazole, propylthiouracil]	Increased concentrations of digoxin.	The clearance of digitalis glycosides may be reduced when a euthyroid state is achieved after the addition of antithyroid agents.
	Thyroid Hormones [levothyroxine, liothyronine, liotrix, thyroid]	Increased concentrations of digoxin.	The clearance of digitalis glycosides may be reduced when a euthyroid state is achieved after the addition of antithyroid agents.
	Verapamil	Increase serum concentration of	Decrease in cardiac glycosides

DRUG	DRUG INTERACTION	EFFECT	MECHANISM OF INTERACTION
		digoxin. Enhance the AV— blocking effect of cardiac glycosides by Calcium channel blockers	clearance by Calcium channel blockers

Epinephrine

DRUG	DRUG INTERACTION	EFFECT	MECHANISM OF INTERACTION
Epinephrine	Beta-Blockers [carteolol, nadolol, penbutolol, pindolol, propranolol, timolol]	Initial hypertensive episode, followed by reflex bradycardia.	Non selective beta blockers unopposed alpha effects and result in vasoconstriction, a subsequent decrease in heart rate occurs due to increased vagal tone(reflex)
	MAO inhibitors[isocarb oxazid, phenelzine, selegiline, tranylcypromine]	Enhance the vasopressor effect of epinephrine (nasal, systemic, oral inhalation)	Inhibition of epinephrine metabolism by MAO inhibition
	Tricyclic antidepressant [amitriptyline, desipramine, doxepin, imipramine,	Enhance the vasopressor effect of epinephrine (nasal, systemic, oral inhalation)	Inhibition of norepinephrine uptake

DRUG	DRUG INTERACTION	EFFECT	MECHANISM OF INTERACTION
	nortriptyline]		

Hydralazine

DRUG	DRUG INTERACTION	EFFECT	MECHANISM OF INTERACTION
Hydralazine	Beta-Blockers (metoprolol, propranolol).	Increased concentrations of both drugs (metoprolol, propranolol).	reduced hepatic blood flow resulting in decreased biotransformation of beta blockers that undergo extensive first-pass metabolism

DIURETICS

Loop Diuretics Bumetanide, Ethacrynic Acid, Furosemide, Torsemide

DRUG	DRUG INTERACTION	EFFECT	MECHANISM OF INTERACTION
Loop Diuretics-class	Aminoglycosides,	Increased risk of auditory toxicity and nephrotoxicity.	Loop Diuretics decrease Aminoglycosides clearance. Increase accumulation of Aminoglycosides in renal tissues
	Cisplatin	Increased risk of ototoxicity and	Additive adverse pharmacologic

DRUG	DRUG INTERACTION	EFFECT	MECHANISM OF INTERACTION
		nephrotoxicity.	effect of the individual agents
	Digoxin,	Increased risk of arrhythmias.	Hypokalemia and possibly hypomagnesemia cased by Loop Diuretics

Furosemide

DRUG	DRUG INTERACTION	EFFECT	MECHANISM OF INTERACTION
Furosemide (See also Loop Diuretics)	Cholestyramine	Decreased GIT absorption of furosemide.	Cholestyramine bind furosemide in GIT that reduce its absorption
	Colestipol	Decreased GI absorption of furosemide.	Colestipol bind furosemide in GIT that reduce its absorption

Thiazide Diuretics

Bendroflumethiazide, Benzthiazide, Chlorothiazide, Chlorthalidone,

Hydrochlorothiazide, Hydroflumethiazide, Indapamide, Methyclothiazide,

Metolazone, Polythiazide, Quinethazone, Trichlormethiazide

DRUG	DRUG INTERACTION	EFFECT	MECHANISM OF INTERACTION
Thiazide Diuretics- class	Digoxin,	Increased risk of arrhythmias.	Hypokalemia and possibly hypomagnesemia cased by Thiazide Diuretics
	Lithium,	Increased concentrations/ toxic effect of lithium.	Decrease renal excretion of lithium
	metformin	Decrease the therapeutic effect of metformin	Hypokalemia induced by thiazide diuretics cause decrease in the effect of metformin
	Sulfonylureas,	Increased fasting blood glucose. Decreased hypoglycemic effects of sulfonylurea.	Thiazide impair insulin sensitivity, increase insulin resistance, increase basal plasma glucose concentration. All of thes may result from hypokalemia produced by Thiazide

Androgens

Nandrolone decanoate

DRUG	DRUG INTERACTION	EFFECT	MECHANISM OF INTERACTION
Nandrolone decanoate	cyclosporine	Nandrolone enhance the hepatotoxic effect of cyclosporine by increasing plasma concentration of cyclosporine	Unknwn, thought to be due to inhibition of hepatic metabolism of cyclosporine
	Warfarin	Increased effects of warfarin.	Androgen— induced increase in antithrombinlll or protein C, or decrease senthesis/ increase destruction of clotting factors

Methyltestosterone/Testosterone

DRUG	DRUG INTERACTION	EFFECT	MECHANISM OF INTERACTION
Methyltestoste rone/ Testosterone	Cyclosporine	Methyltestosteron e/ Testosterone enhance the hepatotoxic effect of cyclosporine by increasing plasma concentration of cyclosporine	Unknwn, thought to be due to inhibition of hepatic metabolism of cyclosporine

DRUG	DRUG INTERACTION	EFFECT	MECHANISM OF INTERACTION
	Warfarin	Increased effects of warfarin.	Androgen—induced increase in antithrombinIII or protein C, or decrease senthesis/increase destruction of clotting factors

ANEMIA DRUGS

Iron Products

Iron Salts (IV)

DRUG	DRUG INTERACTION	EFFECT	MECHANISM OF INTERACTION
Iron Salts (IV) [iron dextran, ferric gluconate, iron sucrose]	ACE inhibitors	ACE inhibitors may enhance the adverse/toxic effect of iron dextran, increase risk of anaphylactic-type reaction	unknown
	Chloramphenicol	reduce the therapeutic efficacy of iron for the treatment of anaemia	decreasing erythropoiesis due to direct bone marrow depression
	dimercaprol	Dimercaprol enhance the nephrotoxic effect	Formation of dimercaprol—iron complex which is

DRUG	DRUG INTERACTION	EFFECT	MECHANISM OF INTERACTION
		of iron salt	more toxic to the kidneys than iron alone

Iron Salts (Oral)

DRUG	DRUG INTERACTION	EFFECT	MECHANISM OF INTERACTION
Iron Salts (Oral) [ferrous fumarate, ferrous gluconate, ferrous sulfate, iron polysaccharide]	Chloramphenicol	reduce the therapeutic efficacy of iron for the treatment of anaemia	decreasing erythropoiesis due to direct bone marrow depression
	cefdinir	Decrease serum concentration of cefdinir. Formation of red-appearing ,non bloody stools may developed due to formation of insoluble iron-cefdinir complex	Formation of insoluble iron-cefdinir complex
	Levodopa	Decreased effects of levodopa.	Formation of poorly absorbed complex
	dimercaprol	Dimercaprol enhance the nephrotoxic effect of iron salt	Formation of dimercaprol—iron complex which is more toxic to the

DRUG	DRUG INTERACTION	EFFECT	MECHANISM OF INTERACTION
			kidneys than iron alone
	Levothyroxine,	Decreased GI absorption of levothyroxine.	Formation of poorly absorbed complex
	methyldopa	Decrease therapeutic effect of methyldopa	Formation of poorly absorbed chelate
	Proton pump inhibitors (esomeprazol, lansoprazole, pantoprazole,rab eprazole)	Decrease serum concentration of iron	Increase in gastrointestinal PH associated with decrease in iron absorption. Also stomach acidity required for releasing iron from dietary sources
	Penicillamine	Decreased GI absorption of penicillamine.	Formation of poorly absorbed chelate
	Antacids[aluminum hydroxide, aluminum-magnesium hydroxide, magnesium hydroxide, sodium bicarbonate]	Decreased GI absorption of iron.	Formation of less foluble iron complexes

DRUG	DRUG INTERACTION	EFFECT	MECHANISM OF INTERACTION
	Quinolones [gatifloxacin, moxifloxacin, sparfloxacin]	Decreased GI absorption of quinolone.	Formation of poorly absorbed chelate
	Tetracyclines,	Decrease serum concentration of tetracycline	Decreased GI absorptionof tetracycline, chelation between tetracycline and iron in GIT.
	Vitamin E	Diminish therapeutic effect of iron salt	unknown

ANTICOAGULANTS/THROMBOLYTIC AGENTS

Alteplase

DRUG	DRUG INTERACTION	EFFECT	MECHANISM OF INTERACTION
Alteplase	Nitroglycerin,	Decreased effects of tPA.	Nitroglycerin increase hepatic blood flow and increase clearance of alteplase
	salicylates [aspirin, bismuth subsalicylate, choline salicylate, magnesium salicylate, salsalate, sodium	Salicylate enhance the adverse/toxic effect of alteplase	Interfering with normal clotting function

DRUG	DRUG INTERACTION	EFFECT	MECHANISM OF INTERACTION
	salicylate, sodium thiosalicylate]		

Dipyridamole

DRUG	DRUG INTERACTION	EFFECT	MECHANISM OF INTERACTION
Dipyridamole	Adenosine	Increased effects of adenosine(profound bradycardia).	Inhibition of adenosine uptake into cells caused by dipyridamole
	Colchicine	Increase serum concentration and adverse/toxic effect of colchicine, increase distribution of colchicines into certain tissue eg. Brain	Inhibition of both p-glycoprotien and CYP3A4 by dipyridamole

Heparin

DRUG	DRUG INTERACTION	EFFECT	MECHANISM OF INTERACTION
Heparin	corticorelin	Significant hypotension and bradycardia	unknown
	nitroglycerin	Decrease serum concentration of	Alteration of antithrombin III

DRUG	DRUG INTERACTION	EFFECT	MECHANISM OF INTERACTION
		heparin. Diminish the anticoagulant effect of heparin	function and chang in heparin concentration by nitroglycerin
	Salicylates [aspirin]	Increased risk of bleeding.	Both drugs possess the potential to cause bleeding

Ticlopidine

DRUG	DRUG INTERACTION	EFFECT	MECHANISM OF INTERACTION
Ticlopidine	clopidogrel	Decrease serum concentration of active metabolite of clopidogrel	CYP2C19 inhibition by Ticlopidine
	Phenytoin,	Increased concentrations of phenytoin.	CYP2C19 inhibition by Ticlopidine
	Theophylline,	Increased concentration of theophylline	Inhibition of CYP1A2 isoenzyme mediated theophylline metabolism by Ticlopidine

Warfarin

DRUG	DRUG INTERACTION	EFFECT	MECHANISM OF INTERACTION
Warfarin	Acetaminophen	Increased effects of warfarin. (if acetaminophen is greater than 1.3 g/day continuously for greater than 1 week)	unknown
	allopurinol	Enhance the anticoagulant effect of warfarin	Inhibition of hepatic warfarin metabolism
	Aminoglutethimide	Decreased effects of warfarin.	Induction of warfarin metabolism by Aminoglutethimide through CYP isoenzymes induction
	Amiodarone	Increased the anticoagulant effects of warfarin.	Inhibition of CYP isoenzymes by amiodarone, and the iodine content of amiodarone may cause hyperthyroidism following chronic use may increase body sensitivity to warfarin
	Androgens[danazol, fluoxymesterone,	Increased effects of warfarin.	Androgen—induced increase in antithrombinIII or

DRUG	DRUG INTERACTION	EFFECT	MECHANISM OF INTERACTION
	methyltestosteron, nandrolone decanoate, oxandrolone, oxymetholone, stanozolol, testosterone]		protein C, or decrease senthesis/ increase destruction of clotting factors
	Azole Antifungals [fluconazole, itraconazole, ketoconazole, miconazole]	Increased effects of warfarin.	Inhibition of CYP3A4 mediated warfarin metabolism by azole Azole Antifungals
	Barbiturates [amobarbital, aprobarbital, butabarbital, butalbital, mephobarbital, pentobarbital, phenobarbital, primidone, secobarbital,	Decreased effects of warfarin.	Induction of CYP isoenzymes mediated warfarin metabolism by Barbiturates
	Carbamazepine	Decreased effects of warfarin.	Induction of warfarin metabolism by Carbamazepine
	Cephalosporins [cefamandole, cefazolin, cefoperazone, cefotetan, cefoxitin, ceftriaxone]	Increased effects of warfarin.	Cephalosporin – associated platelet inhibition. Decrease in gastric normal flora that serve as aminor source of vit. K2

DRUG	DRUG INTERACTION	EFFECT	MECHANISM OF INTERACTION
	Chloramphenicol	Increased effects of warfarin.	Chloramphenicol inhibit the metabolism of phenytoin.
	Chlorpropamide	Increased hypoglycemic effects of chlorpropamide.	possibly by inhibiting Dicumarol hepatic metabolism.
	Cholestyramine	Decreased effects of warfarin.	Cholestyramine bind warfarin in the GI tract both upon initial presentation and during the course of enterohepatic cycle
	Cimetidine	Increased effects of warfarin.	Cimetidine inhibit hepatic metabolism of warfarin (hydroxylation)
	Dextrothyroxine	Increased effects of warfarin	Thyroid hormones increase the catabolism of the clotting factors dependent on vitamin K. The hypoprothrombinemic response to oral anticoagulants may be enhanced
	Disulfiram	Increased effects of warfarin.	Disulfiram inhibit inhibit CYP2C9 isoenzyme

DRUG	DRUG INTERACTION	EFFECT	MECHANISM OF INTERACTION
			mediated S— warfarin metabolism
	Fibric Acids [clofibrate, fenofibrate, gemfibrozil]	Increased effects of warfarin.	1.Fibric Acids cause displacement of warfarin from protein binding sites. 2.Increase affinity of of anticoagulant for binding sites 3. fenofibrate is inhibitor for CYP2C9
	Ginkgo biloba	Enhance the adverse / toxic effect of warfarin	Inhibition of platelet aggregation by Ginkgo biloba increase the effect of warfarin
	Glucagon	Increased effects of warfarin with prolonged glucagon dosing.	unknown
	Glutethimide	Decreased effects of warfarin.	Induction of CYP isoenzyme mediated warfarin metabolism
	Griseofulvin	Decreased effects of warfarin.	Induction of CYP3A4 and CYP2C9 by

DRUG	DRUG INTERACTION	EFFECT	MECHANISM OF INTERACTION
			griseofulvin
	HMG-CoA Reductase Inhibitors [fluvastatin, lovastatin, simvastatin]	Increased effects of warfarin.	Inhibition of CYP2C9 isoenzymes mediated warfarin metabolism
	Levamisole	Increased effects of warfarin.	unknown
	Macrolide Antibiotics [azithromycin, clarithromycin, erythromycin]	Increased effects of warfarin (bleeding tendency).	inhibition of CYP3A4 by Macrolide
	Methyltestosterone/ Testosterone	Increased effects of warfarin.	Androgen— induced increase in antithrombinIII or protein C, or decrease senthesis/ increase destruction of clotting factors
	Metronidazole	Increased effects of warfarin.	Inhibition of CYP2C9 by metronidazole that responsible for S— warfarin metabolism
	Nalidixic Acid	Increased effects of warfarin.	In vitro evidence, Nalidixic Acid is able to diplace warfarin from

DRUG	DRUG INTERACTION	EFFECT	MECHANISM OF INTERACTION
			protein binding site
	NSAIDs [diclofenac, etodolac, fenoprofen, flurbiprofen, ibuprofen, indomethacin, ketoprofen, ketorolac, meclofenamate, nabumetone, naproxen, oxaprozin, piroxicam, sulindac, tolmetin]	Increased effects of warfarin. Increased risk of bleeding.	NSAIDs inhibit platelet aggregation
	Penicillins [ampicillin, dicloxacillin, methicillin, mezlocillin, nafcillin, oxacillin, penicillin G, piperacillin, ticarcillin]	Increased effects of warfarin with large doses of IV penicillin. Nafcillin and dicloxacillin can caus ewarfarin resistance.	Not understood. The nafcillin-warfarin interaction is possibly due to increase in the metabolism of warfarin by the liver. Changes in bleeding times caused by the other penicillins appear to result from changes in antithrombin III activity, blood platelet changes and alterations in the fibrinogen-fibrin conversion.

DRUG	DRUG INTERACTION	EFFECT	MECHANISM OF INTERACTION
			Dicloxacillin possibly reduces serum warfarin levels.
	phenytoin	Increased concentrations of phenytoin. Increased INR and risk of bleeding initially then return to the normal INR.	Inhibition of CYP2C9 mediated phenytoin metabolism by Anticoagulants. Displacement of warfarin from protein binding site by phenytoin initially, then phenytoin induce CYP isoenzymes mediated warfarin metabolism
	Quinine Derivatives [quinidine, quinine]	Enhance the anticoagulant effects of warfarin.	unknown
	Quinolones [ciprofloxacin, enoxacin, norfloxacin]	Increase effect of warfarin	In vitro evidence, quinolones are able to diplace warfarin from protein binding site
	Rifamycins [rifabutin, rifampin, rifapentine]	Decreased effects of warfarin.	Induction of CYP isoenzymes by rifamycins
	Salicylates	Increased effects	inhibit platelet

DRUG	DRUG INTERACTION	EFFECT	MECHANISM OF INTERACTION
	[aspirin, methylsalicylate]	of warfarin with large doses of salicylate. Increased risk of bleeding with any aspirin dose.	aggregation
	sucralfate	Increased effects of warfarin.	Formation of poorly absorbed complex
	Sulfinpyrazone	Increased effects of warfarin.	1.Displacement of warfarin from protein binding sites 2.inhibition of CYP2C9 mediated warfarin metabolism
	Sulfonamides [sulfamethizole, sulfamethoxazole , sulfasalazine, sulfisoxazole, trimethoprim/ sulfamethoxazole]	Increase risk of GIT bleeding (enhanced anticoagulant effect of vit.K antagonists)	1.Displacement of warfarin from protein binding sites 2.sulphonamides associated reduction in GIT flora for vitamine K production 3.sulphonamide inhibit metabolism of warfarin
	Sulfonylureas [acetohexamide,	Increased hypoglycemic	possibly by inhibiting

DRUG	DRUG INTERACTION	EFFECT	MECHANISM OF INTERACTION
	chlorpropamide, glipizide, glyburide, tolazamide, tolbutamide]	effects of tolbutamide.	Dicumarol hepatic metabolism.
	tamoxifen	Increase effect of warfarin	Inhibition of warfarin metabolism by CYP2C9 inhibition
	Thioamines [methimazole, propylthiouracil]	Various effects on warfarin activity.	Antithyroid drugs, by reducing the hyperthyroid state, may increase the hypoprothrombinemic response to oral anticoagulants
	Thyroid Hormones [levothyroxine, liothyronine, liotrix, thyroid]	Increased effects of warfarin.	Thyroid hormones increase the catabolism of the clotting factors dependent on vitamin K. The hypoprothrombinemic response to oral anticoagulants may be enhanced
	Vitamin E (Tocopherol)	Increased effects of warfarin.	Vitamin E interfere with vitamin K— dependant process of clotting factors production
	Vitamin K	Decreased or	Vitamin K interfere

DRUG	DRUG INTERACTION	EFFECT	MECHANISM OF INTERACTION
	(Phytonadione) (food sourse)	reversed effects of warfarin.	with ability of warfarin to inhibit production of clotting factors
	zileuton	Increase effect of R-warfarin	Decrease clearance of R-warfarin

Antiplatelet

Clopidogrel

DRUG	DRUG INTERACTION	EFFECT	MECHANISM OF INTERACTION
Clopidogrel	Acetylsalicylic Acid (aspirin)	prolongation of bleeding time. the risk of gastrointestinal (GI) bleeding may be increased	Clopidogrel has been shown to potentiate the inhibition of platelet aggregation due to aspirin
	clarthromycin	Diminish the therapeutic effect of clopidogrel	inhibition of CYP3A4 by Clarithromycin cause reduction in clopidogrel bioactivation
	delavirdine	Decrease serum concentration of active metabolites of clopidogrel (decrease	Inhibition of CYP2C19 mediated clopidogrel metabolism/ activation

DRUG	DRUG INTERACTION	EFFECT	MECHANISM OF INTERACTION
		effectivity)	
	enoxaparin	potentiate the risk of bleeding complications	Clopidogrel has been shown to potentiate the inhibition of platelet aggregation due to anticoagulants
	esomeprazole	reduce the cardioprotective effects of clopidogrel.	The proposed mechanism is PPI inhibition of the CYP450 2C19-mediated metabolic bioactivation of clopidogrel
	fluconazole	Decrease the active metabolites of clopidogril, decrease platelet inhibition and increase the concentration of (parent) clopidogrel.	CYP2C19 inhibition by fluconazole
	glimepiride	potentiating toxicity of glimepiride	In vitro studies have shown that high concentrations of clopidogrel inhibit CYP450 2C9 isoenzymes
	isoniazid	Decrease serum	Inhibition of

DRUG	DRUG INTERACTION	EFFECT	MECHANISM OF INTERACTION
		concentration of active metabolite of clobidogrel	CYP2C19 by INH
	Proton Pump Inhibitors [esomeprazole, lansoprazole, omeprazole, pantoprazole, rabeprazole]	Coadministration with proton pump inhibitors (PPIs) may reduce the cardioprotective effects of clopidogrel.	The proposed mechanism is PPI inhibition of the CYP450 2C19-mediated metabolic bioactivation of clopidogrel
	Rifamycines	Enhance the therapeutic effects of clopidogrel	CYP3A4 induction cause increase in clopidogrel bioactivation
	SSRIs	Decrease antiplatelet activity and Increase serum concentration of clopidogrel.	CYP2C19 inhibition by SSRIs,decrease serum concentration of active metabolite of clopidogrel
	Ticlopidine	Decrease serum concentration of active metabolite of clopidogrel	CYP2C19 inhibition by Ticlopidine

ANTINEOPLASTIC DRUGS

Azathioprine

DRUG	DRUG INTERACTION	EFFECT	MECHANISM OF INTERACTION
Azathioprine	Allopurinol	Increased effects of Azathioprine	Allopurinol inhibit xanthine oxidase, the enzyme responsible for the first pass metabolism of Azathioprine
	ACE inhibitors	Enhance the neutropenic effect of Azathioprine	Related to the additive toxic effect of individual agents on bone marrow
	Tacrolimus (topical)	Enhance the adverse/ toxic effect of Azathioprine (risk of infection, lymphoma, and skin malignancy	Augmentation of immunosupprssion

Methotrexate

DRUG	DRUG INTERACTION	EFFECT	MECHANISM OF INTERACTION
Methotrexate	digoxin	Decreased concentrations of digoxin.	1.Interference with digoxin tablet dissolution. 2.also possible that

DRUG	DRUG INTERACTION	EFFECT	MECHANISM OF INTERACTION
			intestinal epithelial toxicity plays arole 3. increase hepatic p-glycoprotein
	NSAIDs [diclofenac, etodolac, fenoprofen, flubiprofen, ibuprofen, indomethacin, ketoprofen, ketorolac, meclofenamate, mefenamic acid, nabumetone, naproxen, oxaprozin, piroxicam, sulindac, tolmetin]	Increased risk of methotrexate toxicity.	NSAIDs decrease renal excretion of methotrexate throughout renal prostaglandin senthesis inhibition
	Penicillins[amoxic illin, ampicillin, bacampicillin, carbenicillin, cloxacillin, dicloxacillin, methicillin, mezlocillin, penicillin G, penicillin V, piperacillin, ticarcillin]	Increased concentrations of methotrexate. Increased risk of methotrexate toxicity.	Penicillins are weak acids that compate with methotrexate for excretion sites in the renal tubules
	Probenecid	Increased concentrationsof	compate with methotrexate for

DRUG	DRUG INTERACTION	EFFECT	MECHANISM OF INTERACTION
		methotrexate. Increased risk of methotrexate toxicity.	excretion sites in the renal tubules
	Salicylates [aspirin, bismuth subsalicylate, choline magnesium salicylate, choline salicylate, magnesium salicylate salsalate, sodium salicylate, sodium thiosalicylate	Increased risk of methotrexate toxicity.	1.compate with methotrexate for excretion sites in the renal tubules 2. decrease renal excretion of methotrexate throughout renal prostaglandin senthesis inhibition
	Sulfonamides [sulfadiazine, sulfamethizole, sulfamethoxazole, sulfasalazine, sulfisoxazole, trimethoprim/sul famethoxazole]	Increased risk of bone marrow suppression and megaloblastic anemia.	Both drug cause folate deficiency (suppression of dihydrofolate reductase)
	Theophylline derivatives	Increase effect of theophylline	Decrease in renal excretion of theophylline
	tetracyclins	Increase serum concentration of methotrexate.	suppressing metabolism of the drug by bacteria in GIT

ARTHRITIS AND GOUT AGENTS

Allopurinol

DRUG	DRUG INTERACTION	EFFECT	MECHANISM OF INTERACTION
Allopurinol	Ampicillin	Increased rate of Ampicillin-associated skin rash	Potentiation of Ampicillin effect (not well defined)
	ACE inhibitors	Enhance the potential for allergic or hypersensitivity reactions to allopuranol (stevens-johnson syndrome)	unknown but impaired renal function may be a predisposing factor
	Chlorpropamide	Increase serum concentration of Chlorpropamide	Competition for renal excretion
	didanosine	Increase risk of toxicity of didanosine	Inihibition of didanosine metabolism by inhibition of xanthine oxidase mediated metabolism, or indirectly by accumulation of hypoxanthine phosphorylase-mediated didanosin metabolism

DRUG	DRUG INTERACTION	EFFECT	MECHANISM OF INTERACTION
	Thiopurines [azathioprine, mercaptopurine]	Increased effects of Thiopurines	Allopurinol inhibit xanthine oxidase, the enzyme responsible for the first pass metabolism of Thiopurines
	warfarin	Enhance the anticoagulant effect of warfarin	Inhibition of hepatic warfarin metabolism

Colchicine

DRUG	DRUG INTERACTION	EFFECT	MECHANISM OF INTERACTION
Colchicine	Cyclosporine,	Increased risk of cyclosporine toxicity (GI, hepatic, renal, neuromuscular).	competitive inhibition of P-glycoprotein (P-gp) efflux transporter in the intestine, renal proximal tubule and liver, resulting in increased drug absorption and decreased excretion
	Clarithromycin	Increase serum concentration of colchicines. Colchicines toxicity	inhibition of CYP3A4 by Clarithromycin, and p-glycoprotien –

DRUG	DRUG INTERACTION	EFFECT	MECHANISM OF INTERACTION
		(gastrointestinal symptoms, hematological abnormalities,neuropathies, myopathies	mediated colchicine transport
	dipyridamole	Increase serum concentration and adverse/toxic effect of colchicine, increase distribution of colchicines into certain tissue eg. Brain	Inhibition of both p-glycoprotien and CYP3A4 by dipyridamole
	erythromycin	Increase serum concentration of colchicines. Colchicines toxicity (gastrointestinal symptoms, hematological abnormalities,neuropathies, myopathies	inhibition of CYP3A4 by erythromycin, and p-glycoprotien – mediated colchicine transport
	mtronidazole	Increase serum concentration (increase toxic effect)	CYP3A4 inhibition by mtronidazole
	Tetracycline	Increase serum concentration of colchicines	Tetracycline is moderate CYP3A4 inhibitor

Nonsteroidal Anti-Inflammatory Drugs (NSAIDs)

Diclofenac, Etodolac, Fenoprofen, Flubiprofen, Ibuprofen, Indomethacin, Ketoprofen, Ketorolac, Meclofenamate, Mefenamic Acid, Nabumetone, Naproxen, Piroxicam, Sulindac, Tolmetin

DRUG	DRUG INTERACTION	EFFECT	MECHANISM OF INTERACTION
Nonsteroidal Anti-Inflammatory Drugs (NSAIDs)	Aminoglycosides,	Increased concentrations of aminoglycoside in premature infants.	NSAIDs inhibit cyclooxygenase (COX), an enzyme involved in renal prostaglandin synthesis. This inhibition cause deterioration of glomerular filtration rate
	Angiotensing ConvertingEnzyme Inhibitors [benazepril, captopril, enalapril, fosinopril, lisinopril, moexipril, quinapril, ramipril, trandolapril]	Decreased effects of angiotensin converting enzyme inhibitor.	Effect on vascular tone and fluid homeostasis
	Beta-Blockers	Decreased	Effect on vascular

DRUG	DRUG INTERACTION	EFFECT	MECHANISM OF INTERACTION
		antihypertensive effects of beta-blocker.	tone and fluid homeostasis
	cyclosporine	Enhance the nephrotoxic effect of cyclosporine, and increase serum concentration of cyclosporine	Inhibition of PG synthesis especially in kidney. The mechanism of increase in concentration is unclear
	Lithium	Increased concentrations of lithium.	NSAIDs decrease renal excretion of lithium throughout renal prostaglandin senthesis inhibition
	Methotrexate	Increased risk of methotrexate toxicity.	NSAIDs decrease renal excretion of methotrexate throughout renal prostaglandin senthesis inhibition
	Serotonin Reuptake Inhibitors [fluoxetine, fluvoxamine, paroxetine, sertraline]	Enhance the antiplatelet effect of NSAIDs (GIT bleeding risk)	Inhibition of gastroprotective prostaglandins by both drugs
	Warfarin,	Increased effects of warfarin. Increased risk of	NSAIDs inhibit platelet aggregation

DRUG	DRUG INTERACTION	EFFECT	MECHANISM OF INTERACTION
		bleeding.	

Indomethacin

DRUG	DRUG INTERACTION	EFFECT	MECHANISM OF INTERACTION
Indomethacin *(See also* Nonsteroidal Anti-Inflammatory Drugs (NSAIDs))	Digoxin,	Increased concentrations of digoxin in premature infants.	Decrease in renal perfusion resultfrom inhibition of prostaglandin decrease digoxin clearance

Ketorolac

DRUG	DRUG INTERACTION	EFFECT	MECHANISM OF INTERACTION
Ketorolac *(See also* Nonsteroidal Anti-Inflammatory Drugs (NSAIDs))	Probenecid	Increased risk of ketorolac toxicity.	Decrease in renal excretion of ketorolac by competetion
	Salicylates [aspirin]	Increased risk of ketorolac adverse effects(GI bleeding, renal dysfunction . . .)	Synergistic effect

Naproxen

DRUG	DRUG INTERACTION	EFFECT	MECHANISM OF INTERACTION
Naproxen (See also Nonsteroidal Anti-Inflammatory Drugs (NSAIDs))	tapentadol	Increase serum concentration of tapentadol	Glucuronosyltransf erase (UGT1A9) inhibition by naproxen

Piroxicam

DRUG	DRUG INTERACTION	EFFECT	MECHANISM OF INTERACTION
Piroxicam (See also Nonsteroidal Anti-Inflammatory Drugs (NSAIDs))	Ritonavir	Increased risk of piroxicam toxicity.	Inhibition of CYP 2C9 by Ritonavir

BRONCHODILATORS

Theophyllines Aminophylline, Dyphylline, Oxtriphylline, Theophylline

DRUG	DRUG INTERACTION	EFFECT	MECHANISM OF INTERACTION
Theophyllines-	Acyclovir	Increased	inhibition of

DRUG	DRUG INTERACTION	EFFECT	MECHANISM OF INTERACTION
class		concentrations of theophylline.	theophylline oxidative metabolism
	amiodarone	Increase toxic effect of theophylline	Inhibition of enzymes responsible for theophylline metabolism
	benzodiazepines	Diminish therapeuyic effect of benzodiazepines	Xanthine blockade of adenosine receptors oe xanthine induce metabolism of benzodiazepines
	Barbiturates[amo barbital, aprobarbital, butabarbital, butalbital, mephobarbital, pentobarbital, phenobarbital, primidone, secobarbital]	Decreased concentrations of theophylline.	Induction of CYP1A2 and CYP3A4 mediated theophylline metabolism by barbiturates
	Beta-Blockers, noncardio-selective[carteolo l, penbutolol, pindolol, propranolol, timolol]	Increased concentrations of theophylline. Pharmacologic antagonism may decrease effects of one or both drugs.	Decrease theophylline clearance, inhibition of CYP1A2 and or 3A4 by propranolol mediated theophylline metabolism and antagonism of theophylline effect

DRUG	DRUG INTERACTION	EFFECT	MECHANISM OF INTERACTION
			by beta receptor blocking
	carbamazepine	Decrease the effect of both drugs	Carbamazepine increase clearance of theophylline by induction of CYP1A2, the mechanism by which theophylline effect carbamazepine
	Cimetidine	Increased concentrations of theophylline.	Inhibition of CYP isoenzyme mediated theophylline metabolism
	Contraceptives (estrogen), Oral	Increased concentrations of theophylline.	Contraceptives decrease hepatic clearance of theophylline by inhibiting its metabolism
	Diltiazem	Increased concentrations of theophylline.	Inhibition of CYP3A4 by diltiazem
	Disulfiram	Increased concentrations of theophylline.	Inhibition of CYP isoenzyme mediated theophylline metabolism by Disulfiram
	Halothane	Increased risk of	Halothane

DRUG	DRUG INTERACTION	EFFECT	MECHANISM OF INTERACTION
		arrhythmias.	increases the arrhythmogenic potential of catecholamines. Theophylline appears to enhance the release of catecholamines.
	Hydantoins [fosphenytoin, phenytoin]	Decreased concentrations of theophylline.	Hydantoins induce CYP3A4 isoenzymes.
	Macrolide Antibiotics[azithromycin, clarithromycin, dirithromycin, erythromycin, troleandomycin]	Increased concentrations of theophylline.	Macrolide inhibit CYP3A4 isoenzymes.
	methotrexate	Increase effect of theophylline	Decrease in renal excretion of theophylline
	Mexiletine	Increased concentrations of theophylline	Mexiletine inhibit CYP1A2, the primary metabolizing isoenzyme for theophylline
	Quinolones [ciprofloxacin, enoxacin, norfloxacin]	Increased concentrations of theophylline.	Quinolones inhibit CYP1A2 and/or CYP3A4, mediated metabolism of theophylline

DRUG	DRUG INTERACTION	EFFECT	MECHANISM OF INTERACTION
	Rifamycins [rifabutin, rifampin, rifapentine]	Decreased concentrations of theophylline.	CYP3A4 and CYP1A2 induction by rifamycins
	Thiabendazole	Increased concentrations of theophylline.	Thiabendazole inhibit metabolism of theophylline
	Thioamines [methimazole, propylthiouracil]	Decreased theophylline concentrations in hyperthyroid patients; returns to normal once euthyroid state achieved.	Clearance of theophylline and related agents depends upon thyroid function. In the hyperthyroid state, clearance may be enhanced. In the hypothyroid state, clearance may be reduced. Theophylline clearance may decrease and the risk of toxicity may increase when hyperthyroid patients become euthyroid.
	Thyroid Hormones[dextrothyroxine, levothyroxine, liothyronine, liotrix, thyroglobulin, thyroid]	Decreased theophylline concentrations in hyperthyroid patients; returns to normal once euthyroid state achieved.	Increase in theophylline metabolism in hyperthyroid patients. Decrease theophylline metabolism in

DRUG	DRUG INTERACTION	EFFECT	MECHANISM OF INTERACTION
			hypothyroid patient
	Ticlopidine	Increased concentration of theophylline	Inhibition of CYP1A2 isoenzyme mediated theophylline metabolism by Ticlopidine
	Zileuton	Increased concentration of theophylline.	Zileuton inhibit CYP isoenzyme mediated theophylline metabolism

Leukotriene Inhibitors

Zileuton

DRUG	DRUG INTERACTION	EFFECT	MECHANISM OF INTERACTION
Zileuton	propranolol	Increase effect of propranolol	Increase B—blockage accompanied by concomitant use of these drugs
	Theophylline,	Increased concentration of theophylline.	Zileuton inhibit CYP isoenzyme mediated theophylline metabolism
	R-warfarin	Increase effect of R-warfarin	Decrease clearance of warfarin

ANTIPARKINSON AGENTS

Levodopa

DRUG	DRUG INTERACTION	EFFECT	MECHANISM OF INTERACTION
Levodopa	Hydantoins [ethotoin, fosphenytoin, mephenytoin, phenytoin]	Decreased effects of levodopa.	Hydantoins can alter dopaminergic signaling in the CNS(ie. Decrease in some region and increase in other)
	Iron Salts (Oral) [ferrous fumarate, ferrous gluconate, ferrous sulfate, iron polysaccharide]	Decreased effects of levodopa.	Formation of poorly absorbed complex
	MAO Inhibitors [phenelzine, tranylcypromine]	Increase concentration of levodopa. Increased risk of hypertensive reactions.	MAO Inhibitors involved in inhibition of levodopa metabolism
	methylphenidate	Enhance the adverse/ toxic effect of levodopa	Inhibition of dopamine reuptake by methylphenidate that increase effect of dopamine agonist
	metoclopramide	Decrease therapeutic effect of levodopa	Antidopaminergic effect of metoclopramide decrease the effect of dopamine agonist

DRUG	DRUG INTERACTION	EFFECT	MECHANISM OF INTERACTION
	Pyridoxine	Decrease therapeutic effect of levodopa	Pyridoxine enhance the conversion of levodopa to dopamine, and thus decrase the amount of levodopa available to cross blood-brain barrier to exert its therapeutic effect

ANTICONVULSANTS

Carbamazepine

DRUG	DRUG INTERACTION	EFFECT	MECHANISM OF INTERACTION
Carbamazepine	Bupropion	Decreased effects of bupropion.	Induction of CYP2B6 mediated Bupropion metabolism by carbamazepine
	Cimetidine	Increased concentrations of carbamazepine.	Cimetidine inhibit metabolism (CYP3A4) of carbamazepine and/or effect its absorption
	clarithromycin	Increased concentrations of carbamazepine.	Inhibition of hepatic metabolism of carbamazepine and inhibition of CYP3A4 enzymes

DRUG	DRUG INTERACTION	EFFECT	MECHANISM OF INTERACTION
	Cyclosporine,	Decreased concentrations of cyclosporine.	Induction of CYP3A4 mediated Cyclosporine metabolism by carbamazepine
	Danazol	Increased concentrations of carbamazepine.	Inhibition of CYP3A4 mediated carbamazepine metabolism by Danazol
	Diltiazem	Increased concentrations of carbamazepine. Decrease concentration of Diltiazem	Inhibition of CYP isoenzymes mediated carbamazepine metabolism by Diltiazem. Induction of CYP isoenzymes mediated Diltiazem metabolism
	Doxycycline,	Decreased concentrations of doxycycline.	Incuction of metabolism or excretion of doxycycline by carbamazepine (enzymes and/ or transports is uncertain)
	erythromycin	Increased concentrations of	Inhibition of hepatic

DRUG	DRUG INTERACTION	EFFECT	MECHANISM OF INTERACTION
		carbamazepine.	metabolism of carbamazepine and inhibition of CYP3A4 enzymes
	Felodipine,	Increased concentrations of carbamazepine. Decrease concentration of Felodipine	Inhibition of CYP isoenzymes mediated carbamazepine metabolism by Felodipine. Induction of CYP isoenzymes mediated Felodipine metabolism
	Fluoxetine	Increased concentrations of carbamazepine.	Inhibition of CYP3A4 mediated carbamazepine metabolism by Fluoxetine
	Haloperidol,	Decreased effects of haloperidol.	Induction of CYP isoenzyme mediated haloperidol metabolism by carbamazepine
	Isoniazid	Increased risk of carbamazepine toxicity	Inhibition of CYP isoenzymes mediated carbamazepine metabolism by Isoniazid.

DRUG	DRUG INTERACTION	EFFECT	MECHANISM OF INTERACTION
	Lamotrigine,	Decreased concentrations of lamotrigine. Increased risk of carbamazepine toxicity.	Induction of CYP isoenzyme mediated Lamotrigine metabolism by carbamazepine. Increase in the formation of active metabolite carbamazepine-epoxide
	Lithium,	Increased risk of neurotoxicity (lethargy, muscular weakness, ataxia, tremor, hyperreflexia).	Unknown (no change in serum concentration of any drug)
	Macrolide Antibiotics [clarithromycin, erythromycin, troleandomycin]	Increased concentrations of carbamazepine.	Inhibition of hepatic metabolism of carbamazepine by inhibition of CYP3A4 enzymes
	MAO Inhibitors [isocarboxazid, phenelzine, tranylcypromine]	Increased risk of severe adverse effects of MAO Inhibitors (hyperpyrexia, hyperexcitability, muscle rigidity, seizures).	Carbamazepine altering concentration, metabolism and distribution of many MAO Inhibitors

DRUG	DRUG INTERACTION	EFFECT	MECHANISM OF INTERACTION
	Nefazodone	Increased concentrations of carbamazepine. Decreased concentrations of nefazodone.	Inhibition os CYP3A4 mediated carbamazepine metabolism by Nefazodone. Induction of Nefazodone metabolism by carbamazepine
	Phenytoin,	Decreased concentrations of carbamazepine. Variable effects on concentrations of phenytoin.	Induction of carbamazepine metabolism by Phenytoin. Induction of Phenytoin metabolism by carbamazepine
	Primidone	Decreased concentrations of carbamazepine, primidone, and phenobarbital (metabolite of primidone).	Induction of CYP2C8 isoenzymes by carbamazepine and primidone
	Propoxyphene	Increased concentration and CNS depressant effect of carbamazepine.	Inhibition of CYP3A4 by Propoxyphene. Synergestic CNS depressant effect of both drugs

DRUG	DRUG INTERACTION	EFFECT	MECHANISM OF INTERACTION
	Serotonin Reuptake Inhibitors paroxetine, sertraline]	Increase carbamazepine concentration and decrease concentration of SSRIs	Inhibition of CYP3A4 by SSRIs and induction of CYP1A2,2c,and/or 3A4 by carbamazepine
	Theophylline class	Decrease the effect of both drugs	Carbamazepine increase clearance of theophylline by induction of CYP1A2, the mechanism by which theophylline effect carbamazepine
	Tricyclic Antidepressants [amitriptyline, desipramine, doxepin, imipramine, nortriptyline]	Decreased concentrations of tricyclic antidepressant.	Induction of CYP isoenzyme mediated Tricyclic Antidepressants metabolism by carbamazepine
	Valproic acid	Decreased concentrations of valproic acid.	Induction of CYP2C9, CYP2C19 and glucuronidation mediated valproic acid metabolism by carbamazepine
	Verapamil	Increased concentrations of carbamazepine.	Inhibition of CYP isoenzymes mediated carbamazepine metabolism by

DRUG	DRUG INTERACTION	EFFECT	MECHANISM OF INTERACTION
		Decrease concentration of Verapamil	Verapamil. Induction of CYP isoenzymes mediated Verapamil metabolism
	Warfarin,	Decreased effects of warfarin.	Induction of warfarin metabolism by Carbamazepine

Lamotrigine

DRUG	DRUG INTERACTION	EFFECT	MECHANISM OF INTERACTION
Lamotrigine	Carbamazepine	Decreased concentrations of lamotrigine. Increased risk of carbamazepine toxicity.	Induction of CYP isoenzyme mediated Lamotrigine metabolism by carbamazepine. Increase in the formation of active metabolite carbamazepine-epoxide
	Contraceptives (progestins)	Decrease serum concentration of contraceptives	Lamotrigine-mediated induction of levonorgestrel glucuronidation

DRUG	DRUG INTERACTION	EFFECT	MECHANISM OF INTERACTION
	Valproic Acid [divalproex sodium, valproic acid, valproate sodium]	Increased concentrations/toxic effect of lamotrigine.	Inhibition of glucuronidation mediated lamotrigine metabolism, and inhibition of p-glycoprotein that decrease presentation of lamotrigine to the metabolism site

Phenobarbital

DRUG	DRUG INTERACTION	EFFECT	MECHANISM OF INTERACTION
Phenobarbital	Beta-Blockers [metoprolol, propranolol]	Decreased bioavailability of beta-blocker.	Induction of metabolism that is not excreted unchanged in urine
	Corticosteroids,	Decreased effects of corticosteroid.	Induction of CYP isoenzyme mediated Corticosteroids metabolism by Corticosteroids
	diltiazem	Decrease effect of diltiazem	Inhibition of CYP3A4 isoenzyme by barbiturates
	Doxycycline,	Decreased concentrations of doxycycline.	Incuction of metabolism or excretion of

DRUG	DRUG INTERACTION	EFFECT	MECHANISM OF INTERACTION
			doxycycline by barbiturates (enzymes and/ or transports is uncertain)
	Estrogens,	Decreased concentrations of estrogen (contraceptive failure).	Barbiturates induce metabolism of Estrogens
	Ethanol,	Additive CNS effects including impaired coordination, sedation, and death with acute ethanol ingestion (potentially fatal).	The mechanism is related to inhibition of microsomal enzymes acutely and induction of hepatic microsomal enzymes chronically
	Felodipine,	Decrease effect of Felodipine	induction of CYP3A4 isoenzyme by barbiturates
	Folic acid	Decrease serum concentration of phenobarbital	Inhibition of parahydroxylation of Phenobarbital by folic acid
	Griseofulvin,	Decreased concentrationsof griseofulvin	Decrease absorption of griseofulvin
	Methadone,	Decreased effects of methadone. Possible with— drawal symptoms	Induction of metabolic enzymes mediated Methadone

DRUG	DRUG INTERACTION	EFFECT	MECHANISM OF INTERACTION
		in patients on chronic methadone therapy.	metabolism
	Metronidazole,	Therapeutic failure of metronidazole.	Increase Metronidazole elimination (metabolism of Metronidazole ont affected
	Nifedipine,	Decrease effect of Nifedipine	induction of CYP3A4 isoenzyme by barbiturates
	Quinidine,	Decreased concentrations of quinidine and increase toxic effect (hepatotoxicity) of quinidine	Induction of CYP3A4 and CYP2C9 by barbiturates. Both barbiturates and Quinidine can induce hepatotoxicity
	Theophylline,	Decreased concentrations of theophylline.	Induction of CYP1A2 and CYP3A4 mediated theophylline metabolism by barbiturates
	Valproic Acid	Increased concentrations of barbiturate. Decrease concentration of	Inhibition of CYP2C9, N-glucosidation and o-glucuronidation of barbiturate by Valproic Acid.

DRUG	DRUG INTERACTION	EFFECT	MECHANISM OF INTERACTION
		Valproic Acid	Barbiturate induce CYP-mediated oxidation of Valproic Acid
	Voriconazole,	Decreased concentrations of voriconazole. therapy failure	Induction of metablizing enzymes for Voriconazole by Barbiturate
	Warfarin,	Decreased effects of warfarin.	Induction of CYP metablizing enzymes for Warfarin by Barbiturate

Hydantoins [ethotoin, fosphenytoin, mephenytoin, phenytoin]

DRUG	DRUG INTERACTION	EFFECT	MECHANISM OF INTERACTION
Hydantoins [ethotoin, fosphenytoin, mephenytoin, phenytoin]	Amiodarone	Increased concentrations of Hydantoins. Decreased concentrations of amiodarone.	Inhibition of CYP2C9 mediated hydantoin metabolism by amiodarone. CYP isenzyme induction by Hydantoins
	acetaminophen	Increased risk of acetaminophen-induced hepatotoxicity.	Induction of CYP and UDPGTase isoenzyme mediated acetaminophen metabolism.

DRUG	DRUG INTERACTION	EFFECT	MECHANISM OF INTERACTION
			Formation of acetaminophen metabolites which exceed glutathione binding capacity
	Anticoagulants [anisidione, dicumarol, warfarin]	Increased concentrations of Hydantoins. Increased INR and risk of bleeding initially then return to the normal INR.	Inhibition of CYP2C9 mediated Hydantoins metabolism by Anticoagulants. Displacement of warfarin from protein binding site by Hydantoins initially, then Hydantoins induce CYP isoenzymes mediated warfarin metabolism
	Carbamazepine	Decreased concentrations of carbamazepine. Variable effects on concentrations of Hydantoins.	Induction of carbamazepine metabolism by Hydantoins. Induction of Hydantoins metabolism by carbamazepine
	calcium channel blockers	Increase Hydantoins toxicity	calcium channel blockers may effect Hydantoins clearance, either by CYP3A4 inhibition or

DRUG	DRUG INTERACTION	EFFECT	MECHANISM OF INTERACTION
			by change in hepatic blood flow
	Chloramphenicol	Increased concentrations of Hydantoins (three fold). Variable effects on concentrations of chloramphenicol.	Chloramphenicol inhibit the metabolism of Hydantoins.
	Cimetidine	Increased concentrations of Hydantoins.	Inhibition of CYP isoenzyme mediated
	Ciprofloxacin	Decrease serum concentration of Hydantoins. Patient experience seizure	The mechanism is unclear. Animal data indicate change in renal excretion of Hydantoins. Ciprofloxacin alone can cause seizure
	Corticosteroids [betamethasone, cortisone, desoxycorticoster one, dexamethasone, fludrocortisone, hydrocortisone,	Decreased effects of corticosteroid.	induce the CYP450 3A4 hepatic metabolism of corticosteroids and increase their clearance and decrease their half-lives

DRUG	DRUG INTERACTION	EFFECT	MECHANISM OF INTERACTION
	methylprednisolone, paramethasone, prednisolone, prednisone, triamcinolone]		
	Cyclosporine,	Decreased concentrations of cyclosporine.	CYP3A4 induction by Hydantoins
	Diazoxide	Decreased concentrations of Hydantoins.	Diazoxide displace Hydantoins from protein binding site together with increase in renal clearance of Hydantoins
	Disopyramide,	Decreased concentrationsof disopyramide. Increased risk of anticholinergic effects.	CYP3A4 induction by Hydantoins
	Disulfiram	Increased concentrations of Hydantoins.	Decrease Hydantoins metabolism and clearance by inhibition of CYP2C9 the primary pathway for Hydantoins metabolism

DRUG	DRUG INTERACTION	EFFECT	MECHANISM OF INTERACTION
	Dopamine	Increased risk of profound hypotension and cardiac arrest.	unknown
	Doxycycline,	Decreased concentrations of doxycycline.	Incuction of metabolism or excretion of doxycycline by Hydantoins (enzymes and/ or transports is uncertain)
	Estrogens [conjugated estrogens, esterified estrogens, estradiol, estrone, estropipate, esthinyl estradiol, mestranol],	Decreased concentrations of estrogen.	Hydantoins induce metabolism of Estrogens
	Felbamate	Increased concentrations of phenytoin. Decreased concentrations of felbamate.	Inhibition of phenytoin metabolism by Felbamate. Induction of CYP mediated metabolism of Felbamate by phenytoin
	Fluconazole	Increased	Inhibition of CYP2C9

DRUG	DRUG INTERACTION	EFFECT	MECHANISM OF INTERACTION
		concentrations of phenytoin.	by Fluconazole
	Fluoxetine	Increased concentrations of phenytoin.	Inhibition of CYP2C9 by Fluoxetine
	Folic acid	Decreased concentrations of phenytoin.	Folic acid is a cofactor for phenytoin metabolism thus high Folic acid can increase in affinity of phenytoin to metabolizing enzymes
	Isoniazid	Increased concentrations of phenytoin.	Isoniazid inhibit CYP2C19, CYP2C9 and CYP3A4 mediated phenytoin metabolism
	Itraconazole,	Decreased effects of itraconazole. Increased effects of hydantoin.	Inhibition of CYP2C9 by itraconazole
	ketoconazole	Decreased effects of ketoconazole. Increase serum concentration of Hydantoins	Induction of CYP3A4 by Hydantoins that mediated metabolism of ketoconazole. Inhibition of CYP2C9 and or CYP2C19 mediated metabolism of

DRUG	DRUG INTERACTION	EFFECT	MECHANISM OF INTERACTION
			Hydantoins by azole antifungal
	Levodopa,	Decreased effects of levodopa.	Hydantoins can alter dopaminergic signaling in the CNS(ie. Decrease in some region and increase in other)
	Methadone,	Decreased effects of methadone. Possible with-drawal symptoms in patientson chronic methadone therapy.	Induction of hepat metabolism of methadone by Hydantoins
	metronidazole	Metronidazole increase concentration of phenytoin, phenytoin decrease serum concentration of metronidazol	Metronidazole inhibit one or more of the enzymes responsible for phenytoin metabolism, phenytoin induce metronidazole metabolism
	Metyrapone,	Decreased pituitary-adrenal response to metyrapone.	Induction of metyrapone metabolism
	Mexiletine,	Decreased concentrationsof mexiletine.	CYP3A4 induction by Hydantoins

DRUG	DRUG INTERACTION	EFFECT	MECHANISM OF INTERACTION
	Nisoldipine,	Increase phenytoin toxicity	calcium channel blockers may effect phenytoin clearance, either by CYP3A4 inhibition or by change in hepatic blood flow
	Primidone	Increased concentrations of primidone-metabolite (Phenobarbital) Phenobarbital toxicity may produced.	Phenytoin induce Primidone metabolism to produce Phenobarbital and Phenytoin compate with Phenobarbital for the site of metabolism
	Quinidine,	Decreased concentrations/ therapeutic effect of quinidine.	Induction of CYP3A4 and CYP2C9 by Hydantoins
	Rifamycins [rifabutin, rifampin]	Decreased concentrations of phenytoin.	CYP isoenzyme induction of rifamycins
	Sertraline	Increased concentrations of phenytoin	Inhibition of CYP2C9 mediated metabolism of phenytoin by Sertraline
	Sucralfate	reduce phenytoin therapeutic effect	Sucralfate may interfere with the absorption of oral

DRUG	DRUG INTERACTION	EFFECT	MECHANISM OF INTERACTION
			phenytoin
	Sulfonamides [sulfadiazine, sulfamethizole]	Increased concentrations of phenytoin.	Sulfonamides inhibit CYP isoenzyme mediated phenytoin metabolism
	Tacrolimus,	Decreased concentrations of tacrolimus. Increased concentrations of phenytoin.	Induction of CYP3A4 mediated tacrolimus metabolism by phenytoin. The mechanism of increase phenytoin concentration is unclear
	Theophylline,	Decreased concentrations of theophylline.	Hydantoins induce CYP3A4 isoenzymes.
	Ticlopidine	Increased concentrations of phenytoin.	CYP2C19 inhibition by Ticlopidine
	Trimethoprim	Increased concentrations of phenytoin.	Inhibition of CYP isoenzymes by Trimethoprim
	Valproic Acid [divalproex sodium, valproic acid]	Increased concentrations of phenytoin. Decreased concentrations of valproic acid.	Valproic Acid initially displacing phenytoin from protein binding then inhibition CYP mediated phenytoin metabolism. Induction of CYP and

DRUG	DRUG INTERACTION	EFFECT	MECHANISM OF INTERACTION
			UGTS mediated valproate metabolism

Valproic Acid [divalproex sodium, sodium valproate, valproic acid]

DRUG	DRUG INTERACTION	EFFECT	MECHANISM OF INTERACTION
Valproic Acid [divalproex sodium, sodium valproate, valproic acid]	Barbiturates [phenobarbital, primidone]	Increased concentrations of barbiturate. Decrease concentration of Valproic Acid	Inhibition of CYP2C9, N-glucosidation and o-glucuronidation of barbiturate by Valproic Acid. Barbiturate induce CYP-mediated oxidation of Valproic Acid
	Carbamazepine	Decreased concentrations of valproic acid.	Induction of CYP2C9, CYP2C19 and glucuronidation mediated valproic acid metabolism by carbamazepine
	Cholestyramine	Decreased therapeutic effect of valproic acid.	Cholestyramine may interfere with the gastrointestinal absorption of valproic acid reducing serum concentrations, bioavailability and therapeutic effect

DRUG	DRUG INTERACTION	EFFECT	MECHANISM OF INTERACTION
	Felbamate	Increased concentrations of valproic acid.	Felbamate inhibit CYP2C19 mediated valproic acid metabolism
	Lamotrigine,	Increased concentrations/toxic effect of lamotrigine.	Inhibition of glucuronidation mediated lamotrigine metabolism, and inhibition of p-glycoprotein that decrease presentation of lamotrigine to the metabolism site
	Phenytoin,	Increased concentrations of phenytoin. Decreased concentrations of valproic acid.	Valproic Acid initially displacing phenytoin from protein binding then inhibition CYP mediated phenytoin metabolism. Induction of CYP and UGTS mediated valproate metabolism
	rifamycins	Decrease serum concentration of valproic acid	CYP2C19 and CYP2C9 induction of rifamycins
	Salicylates [aspirin, bismuth subsalicylate, choline salicylate,	Increased free (unbound) concentrations of valproic acid.	Protein binding displacement

DRUG	DRUG INTERACTION	EFFECT	MECHANISM OF INTERACTION
	magnesium salicylate, salsalate, sodium salicylate, sodium thiosalicylate]		
	Tricyclic Antidepressants [amitriptyline, desipramine, doxepin, imipramine, nortriptyline]	Increased concentrations of tricyclic antidepressant. Increased risk of serotonin syndrome (CNS irritability,shivering, myoclonus, altered consciousness).	Inhibition of Tricyclic Antidepressants metabolism by valproic acid.

Bupropion

DRUG	DRUG INTERACTION	EFFECT	MECHANISM OF INTERACTION
Bupropion	Carbamazepine	Decreased effects of bupropion.	Induction of CYP2B6 mediated Bupropion metabolism by carbamazepine
	MAO Inhibitors [phenelzine, tranylcypromine]	Increased risk of acute bupropion toxicity (seizures).	Increase in dopamine activity (bupropion inhibit uptake and MAOI Inhibiting the metabolism of dopamine

DRUG	DRUG INTERACTION	EFFECT	MECHANISM OF INTERACTION
	tamoxifen	Reduce clinical effectiveness of tamoxifen	Inhibition of CYP2D6 by bupropion that reduce the formation of highly potent active metabolites of tamoxifen
	Ritonavir	decrease bupropion concentration.	Induction of CYP2B6 mediated bupropion metabolism by Ritonavir

Lithium

DRUG	DRUG INTERACTION	EFFECT	MECHANISM OF INTERACTION
Lithium	amphetamines	Decrease the stimulitary effect of amphetamines	The ability of levodopa to eliminate the lithium-attenuation effect together with less evidence mediated vby dopamine
	Angiotensing Converting Enzyme Inhibitors [benazepril, captopril, enalapril, fosinopril,	Increased concentrations of lithium.	unknown

DRUG	DRUG INTERACTION	EFFECT	MECHANISM OF INTERACTION
	lisinopril, moexipril, quinapril, ramipril, trandolapril]		
	Angiotensin II Receptor Blockers [candesartan, eprosartan, irbesartan, losartan, olmesartan, telmisartan, valsartan]	Increased concentrations of lithium.	Decrease renal elimination of Lithium
	Carbamazepine	Increased risk of neurotoxicity (lethargy, muscular weakness, ataxia, tremor, hyperreflexia).	Unknown (no change in serum concentration of any drug)
	desmopressin	Decrease therapeutic effect of desmopressin. Increase serum concentration of lithium	Decrease translocation of AQP2 (vasoppressin –regulated water channel aquaporin-2) from the cytoplasm that reduce the water reabsorption. Desmopressin decrease renal excretion of lithium
	Haloperidol,	Alterations in consciousness,	unknown

DRUG	DRUG INTERACTION	EFFECT	MECHANISM OF INTERACTION
		encephalopathy, extrapyramidal effects, fever, leukocytosis, and increased serum enzymes.	
	Iodide Salts [calcium iodide, hydrogen iodide, iodide, iodinated glycerol, iodine, potassium iodide, sodium iodide]	Increased risk of hypothyroidism.\n\nEnhance adverse/ toxic effect of lithium	Lithium and Iodide Salts can diminish thyroid function.\n\nLithium block the release of thyroid hormones
	methyldopa	Increase toxic effect of lithium without change in serum concentration of lithium	unknown
	NSAIDs [diclofenac, ibuprofen, indomethacin, ketorolac, meloxicam, naproxen, piroxicam, sulindac]	Increased concentrations of lithium.	NSAIDs decrease renal excretion of methotrexate throughout renal prostaglandin senthesis inhibition
	Sibutramine,	Increased risk of serotonin syndrome (CNS irritability, shivering, myoclonus, altered	Sibutramine inhibit serotonin reuptake and litium have serotonin agonist

DRUG	DRUG INTERACTION	EFFECT	MECHANISM OF INTERACTION
		consciousness).	
	Thiazide Diuretics [bendroflumethiazide, benzthiazide, chlorothiazide, chlorthalidone, hydrochlorothiazide, hydroflumethiazide indapamide, meloxicam, methyclothiazide, metolazone, polythiazide, quinethazone, sulindac, trichlormethiazide	Increased concentrations/ toxic effect of lithium.	Decrease renal excretion of lithium
	Urinary Alkalinizers [potassium citrate, sodium acetate, sodium	Decreased concentrations of lithium.	Urinary Alkalinizers enhance renal excretion of lithium

DRUG	DRUG INTERACTION	EFFECT	MECHANISM OF INTERACTION
	bicarbonate, sodium citrate, sodium lactate, tromethamine]		

SEDATIVES/HYPNOTICS/AGENTS

ANTIDEPRESSANTS:

Monoamine Oxidase Inhibitors(MAO Inhibitors):
Isocarboxazid, Phenelzine, Selegiline, Tranylcypromine

DRUG	DRUG INTERACTION	EFFECT	MECHANISM OF INTERACTION
Monoamine Oxidase (MAO) Inhibitors	Buproprion,	Increased risk of acute bupropion toxicity (seizures).	Increase in dopamine activity (bupropion inhibit uptake and MAOI Inhibiting the metabolism of dopamine
	Carbamazepine,	Increased risk of severe adverse effects of MAO Inhibitors (hyperpyrexia, hyperexcitability, muscle rigidity, seizures).	Carbamazepine altering concentration, metabolism and distribution of many MAO Inhibitors
	dextromethorpha	Enhance the	Increase serotonin

DRUG	DRUG INTERACTION	EFFECT	MECHANISM OF INTERACTION
	n	effect of dextromethorphan (cause serotonin syndrome)	activity during concomitant use
	epinephrine	Enhance the vasopressor effect of epinephrine (nasal, systemic, oral inhalation)	Inhibition of epinephrine metabolism by MAO inhibition
	Insulin,	Increased hypoglycemic effects of insulin.	stimulating insulin secretion
	Levodopa,	Increase concentration of levodopa. Increased risk of hypertensive reactions.	MAO Inhibitors involved in inhibition of levodopa metabolism
	methyldopa	Enhance adverse/toxic effect of methyldopa	involve excessive sympathetic stimulation in the central nervous system.
	Meperidine,	Agitation, seizures, diaphoresis and fever. May progress to coma, apnea, and death.	Additive effect on serotonin, Meperidine block its reuptake and MAOI reduce its metabolism

DRUG	DRUG INTERACTION	EFFECT	MECHANISM OF INTERACTION
	Serotonin Reuptake Inhibitors	Increased risk of serotonin syndrome (CNS irritability, shivering, myoclonus, altered consciousness).	Additive effect on serotonin, Meperidine block its reuptake and MAOI reduce its metabolism
	Sibutramine,	Increased risk of serotonin syndrome (CNS irritability, shivering, myoclonus, altered consciousness).	Sibutramine inhibit serotonin reuptake. MAOI reduce serotonin metabolism
	Sulfonylureas,	Increased hypoglycemic effects of sulfonylurea.	MAO Inhibitors increase the risk of hypoglycemia by enhancing insulin sensitivity
	Tricyclic Antidepressants	Hyperpyretic crisis, seizures. May progress to death.	unknown

Serotonin Reuptake Inhibitors

Citolapram, Escitalopram, Fluoxetine, Fluvoxamine, Nefazodone, Paroxetine, Sertraline, Venlafaxine

DRUG	DRUG INTERACTION	EFFECT	MECHANISM OF INTERACTION
Serotonin Reuptake Inhibitors	carbamazepine	Increased concentrations of carbamazepine.	Inhibition of CYP3A4 mediated carbamazepine metabolism
	cimetidine	Increase serum concentration of SSRIs	CYP3A4 inhibition by cimetidine
	Clozapine	Increased concentrations of clozapine.	SSRIs inhibit CYP isoenzymes mediated Clozapine metabolism
	clopidogrel	Decrease antiplatelet activity and Increase serum concentration of clopidogrel.	CYP2C19 inhibition by SSRIs,decrease serum concentration of active metabolite of clopidogrel
	Cyclosporine	Increased concentrations of cyclosporine.	Inhibition of CYP3A4 mediated cyclosporine metabolism by SSRIs
	Cyproheptadine	Decreased antidepressant effects of serotonin reuptake	Cyproheptadine can cause CNS depression as the most important side effect

DRUG	DRUG INTERACTION	EFFECT	MECHANISM OF INTERACTION
		inhibitor.	
	dronedarone	QTc-prolongation	Both drugs cause prolongation in QTc
	MAO Inhibitors [isocarboxazid, phenelzine, selegiline, tranylcypromine]	Increased risk of serotonin syndrome (CNS irritability, shivering, myoclonus, altered consciousness).	Additive effect on serotonin, Meperidine block its reuptake and MAOI reduce its metabolism
	NSAIDs [diclofenac, ibuprofen, indomethacin, ketorolac, meloxicam, naproxen, piroxicam, sulindac]	Enhance the antiplatelet effect of NSAIDs (GIT bleeding risk)	Inhibition of gastroprotective prostaglandins by both drugs
	Sibutramine,	Increased risk of serotonin syndrome (CNS irritability, shivering, myoclonus, altered consciousness).	Additive effect on serotonin, Sibutramine inhibit serotonin reuptake that increase
	Sympathomimetics [amphetamine, benzphetamine, dextroamphetamine,	Increased risk of serotonin syndrome (CNS irritability, shivering,	Additive effect on serotonin, Sympathomimetics cause adrenergic excess and have

DRUG	DRUG INTERACTION	EFFECT	MECHANISM OF INTERACTION
	dexfenfluramine, diethylpropion, fenfluramine, mazindol, methamphetamin, phendimetrazine, phenmetrazine, phentermine]	myoclonus, altered consciousness).	serotonergic effect
	Tricyclic Antidepressants	Increased concentrations of tricyclic antidepressant. Increased risk of serotonin syndrome (CNS irritability, shivering, myoclonus, altered consciousness).	SSRIs inhibit CYP2D6, CYP1A2, and CYP2C19 mediated Tricyclic Antidepressants metabolism
	quinine	QTc—prolongation	Both drugs cause QTc—prolongation

Fluoxetine

DRUG	DRUG INTERACTION	EFFECT	MECHANISM OF INTERACTION
Fluoxetine

(See also Serotonin Reuptake Inhibitors) | Carbamazepine, | Increased concentrations of carbamazepine. | Inhibition of CYP3A4 mediated carbamazepine metabolism by Fluoxetine |

DRUG	DRUG INTERACTION	EFFECT	MECHANISM OF INTERACTION
	Phenytoin,	Increased concentrations of phenytoin.	Inhibition of CYP2C9 by Fluoxetine
	Thioridazine	Increased risk of cardiac arrhythmias, including ' torsades depointes	Both drugs cause QTc—prolongation

Fluvoxamine

DRUG	DRUG INTERACTION	EFFECT	MECHANISM OF INTERACTION
Fluvoxamine (See also Serotonin Reuptake Inhibitors)	Methadone,	Increased concentrations of methadone.	Fluvoxamine inhibit CYP2C9, CYP2D6, CYP3A4 mediated Methadone metabolism
	phenytoin	Increased concentrations of phenytoin	Inhibition of CYP2C9 mediated metabolism of phenytoin by Sertraline
	Tacrine	Increased concentrations of tacrine.	inhibition of CYP450 1A2 metabolism by fluvoxamine.

DRUG	DRUG INTERACTION	EFFECT	MECHANISM OF INTERACTION
	Thioridazine,	Increased risk of cardiac arrhythmias, including torsades de pointes.	Both drugs cause QTc—prolongation

Paroxetine

DRUG	DRUG INTERACTION	EFFECT	MECHANISM OF INTERACTION
Paroxetine *(See also Serotonin Reuptake Inhibitors)*	Desipramine,	Increased concentrations of tricyclic antidepressant. Increased risk of serotonin syndrome (CNS irritability, shivering, myoclonus, altered consciousness).	The proposed mechanism is paroxetine inhibition of CYP450 2D6, the isoenzyme responsible for the metabolic clearance of many antidepressant and psychotropic drugs
	Imipramine,	Increased concentrations of tricyclic antidepressant. Increased risk of serotonin syndrome (CNS irritability, shivering, myoclonus, altered consciousness).	The proposed mechanism is paroxetine inhibition of CYP450 2D6, the isoenzyme responsible for the metabolic clearance of many antidepressant and psychotropic drugs

DRUG	DRUG INTERACTION	EFFECT	MECHANISM OF INTERACTION
	Phenothiazines,	Increased effects of phenothiazine. Increased risk of life-threatening cardiac arrhythmias with thioridazine.	Both drugs cause QTc—prolongation
	phenytoin	Increased concentrations of phenytoin	Inhibition of CYP2C9 mediated metabolism of phenytoin by Sertraline

Sertraline

DRUG	DRUG INTERACTION	EFFECT	MECHANISM OF INTERACTION
Sertraline (See also Serotonin Reuptake Inhibitors)	Phenytoin,	Increased concentrations of phenytoin	Inhibition of CYP2C9 mediated metabolism of phenytoin by Sertraline
	disulfiram	Enhance the toxic / adverse effect of sertraline	Accumulation of acetaldehyde

Tricyclic Antidepressants (TCAs)

DRUG	DRUG INTERACTION	EFFECT	MECHANISM OF INTERACTION
Tricyclic Antidepressant s-class [amitriptyline, desipramine, doxepin, imipramine, nortriptyline]	Carbamazepine,	Decreased concentrations of tricyclic antidepressant.	Induction of CYP isoenzyme mediated Tricyclic Antidepressants metabolism by carbamazepine
	Cimetidine	Increased concentrations of tricyclic antidepressant.	Inhibition of CYP2C19 mediated tricyclic antidepressant metabolism by Cimetidine
	Clonidine,	Loss of blood pressure control. Increased risk of hypertensive crisis.	tricyclic antidepressant have ability to enhance the pressor response to catecholamines
	Serotonin Reuptake Inhibitors [fluoxetine, fluvoxamine, paroxetine, sertraline]	Increased concentrations of tricyclic antidepressant. Increased risk of serotonin syndrome (CNS irritability, shivering, myoclonus, altered consciousness).	SSRIs inhibit CYP2D6, CYP1A2, and CYP2C19 mediated Tricyclic Antidepressants metabolism

DRUG	DRUG INTERACTION	EFFECT	MECHANISM OF INTERACTION
	MAO Inhibitors [phenelzine, tranylcypromine]	Hyperpyretic crisis, seizures. May progress to death.	unknown
	Rifamycins [rifabutin, rifampin]	Decreased therapeutic effects of tricyclic antidepressant.	Induction of CYP isoenzymes by rifampinycins
	Sparfloxacin	Increased risk of cardiac arrhythmias, including torsades de pointes.	Enhance the QTc-prolongatoion for each drug.
	Sympathomimetics [dobutamine, dopamine, ephedrine, epinephrine, mephentermine, metaraminol, methoxamine, norepinephrine, phenylephrine]	Increased pressor effects of direct-acting sympathomimetics. Decreased pressor effects of indirect-acting sympathomimetics.	TCA inhibition of norepinephrine reuptake in adrenergic neurons, resulting in increased stimulation of adrenergic receptors
	Valproic Acid [divalproex, valproate sodium, valproic acid]	Increased concentrations of tricyclic antidepressant. Increased risk of serotonin syndrome (CNS irritability,	Inhibition of Tricyclic Antidepressants metabolism by valproic acid.

DRUG	DRUG INTERACTION	EFFECT	MECHANISM OF INTERACTION
		shivering, myoclonus, altered consciousness).	

lithium

DRUG	DRUG INTERACTION	EFFECT	MECHANISM OF INTERACTION
Lithium	Angiotensing ConvertingEnzyme Inhibitors [benazepril, captopril, enalapril, fosinopril, lisinopril, moexipril, quinapril, ramipril, trandolapril]	Increased concentrations/toxicity of lithium.	unknown
	Angiotensin II ReceptorBlockers [candesartan, eprosartan, irbesartan, losartan, olmesartan, telmisartan, valsartan]	Increased concentrationsof lithium.	Decrease renal elimination of Lithium
	Carbamazepine	Increased risk of neurotoxicity (lethargy, muscular	Unknown (no change in serum concentration of any drug)

DRUG	DRUG INTERACTION	EFFECT	MECHANISM OF INTERACTION
		weakness, ataxia, tremor, hyperreflexia).	
	Haloperidol,	Alterations in consciousness, encephalopathy, extrapyramidal effects, fever, leukocytosis, and increased serum enzymes.	unknown
	Iodide Salts [calcium iodide, hydrogen iodide, iodide, iodinated glycerol, iodine, potassium iodide, sodium iodide]	Increased risk of hypothyroidism.	Lithium and iodide diminish thyroid function. Lithium block the release of thyroid hormones, iodide interrupts its production
	NSAIDs[diclofenac, ibuprofen, indomethacin, ketorolac, meloxicam, naproxen, piroxicam, sulindac]	Increased concentrations of lithium.	NSAIDs decrease renal excretion of lithium throughout renal prostaglandin senthesis inhibition
	Sibutramine,	Increased risk of serotonin syndrome (CNS irritability, shivering, myoclonus, altered	Sibutramine inhibit serotonin reuptake and litium have serotonin agonist

DRUG	DRUG INTERACTION	EFFECT	MECHANISM OF INTERACTION
		consciousness).	
	Thiazide Diuretics [bendroflumethiazide, benzthiazide, chlorothiazide, chlorthalidone, hydrochlorothiazide, hydroflumethiazide

indapamide, meloxicam,

methyclothiazide,

metolazone, polythiazide,

quinethazone, sulindac,

trichlormethiazide] | Increased concentrations/ toxic effect of lithium. | Decrease renal excretion of lithium |
| | Urinary Alkalinizers [potassium citrate, sodiumacetate, sodium bicarbonate, sodium citrate, sodiumlactate, tromethamine] | Decreased concentrations of lithium. | Increase renal excretion of lithium |

SEDATIVES

Barbiturates Amobarbital, Aprobarbital, Butabarbital, Butalbital, Mephobarbital, Pentobarbital, Phenobarbital, Primidone, Secobarbital

DRUG	DRUG INTERACTION	EFFECT	MECHANISM OF INTERACTION
Barbiturates	Beta-Blockers	Decreased bioavailability of beta-blocker.	Induction of metabolism that is not excreted unchanged in urine
	carbamazepine	Decreased concentrations of carbamazepine, Barbiturates, and phenobarbital (metabolite of Barbiturates).	Induction of CYP2C8 isoenzymes by carbamazepine and Barbiturates
	Corticosteroids [betamethasone, cortisone, desoxycorticosterone, dexamethasone, fludrocortisone, hydrocortisone, methylprednisolone, paramethasone,	Decreased effects of corticosteroid.	Induction of CYP isoenzyme mediated Corticosteroids metabolism by Corticosteroids

DRUG	DRUG INTERACTION	EFFECT	MECHANISM OF INTERACTION
	prednisolone, prednisone, triamcinolone]		
	chloramphenicol	chloramphenicol Increase serum concentration of barbiturates. Barbiturates decrease serum concentration of chloramphenicol	Chloramphenicol diminish barbiturates metabolism. Barbiturates inhibit CYP isoenzymes responsible for chloramphenicol metabolism
	Doxycycline,	Decreased concentrations of doxycycline.	Incuction of metabolism or excretion of doxycycline by barbiturates (enzymes and/ or transports is uncertain)
	diltiazem	Decreased effects of diltiazem	induction of CYP3A4 isoenzyme by barbiturates
	Estrogens [chlorotrianisene, conjugated estrogens, diethylstilbesterol,	Decreased concentrations of estrogen (contraceptive failure).	Barbiturates induce metabolism of Estrogens

DRUG	DRUG INTERACTION	EFFECT	MECHANISM OF INTERACTION
	esterified estrogens, estradiol, estrone, estropipate, ethinyl estradiol,quinestrol		
	Ethanol	CNS depression (potentially fatal).	Additive CNS effects with acute ethanol ingestion
	Felodipine	Decreased effects of felodipine.	induction of CYP3A4 isoenzyme by barbiturates
	Griseofulvin	Decreased concentrationsof griseofulvin	Decrease absorption of griseofulvin
	Methadone	Decreased effects of methadone. Possible with—drawal symptoms in patients on chronic methadone therapy.	Induction of metabolic enzymes mediated Methadone metabolism
	Metronidazole	Therapeutic failure of metronidazole.	Barbiturates increase elimination of metronidazole

DRUG	DRUG INTERACTION	EFFECT	MECHANISM OF INTERACTION
	Nifedipine	Decreased effects of nifedipine.	induction of CYP3A4 isoenzyme by barbiturates
	Quinidine	Decreased concentrations of quinidine	induction of CYP3A4 and possibly CYP2D6 by Barbiturates
	Rifamycins	Rifampin may decrease the plasma concentrations of barbiturates	inducing hepatic metabolism by Rifampin
	Theophyllines,	Decreased concentrations of theophylline.	Induction of CYP1A2 and CYP3A4 mediated theophylline metabolism by barbiturates
	Voriconazole	Decreased concentrations of voriconazole. therapy failure	Induction of metablizing enzymes for Voriconazole by Barbiturate
	Warfarin,	Decreased effects of warfarin.	Induction of CYP isoenzymes mediated warfarin metabolism by Barbiturates
Primidone (See also Barbiturates)	Phenytoin	Increased concentrations of primidone-metabolite	Phenytoin induce Primidone metabolism to produce

DRUG	DRUG INTERACTION	EFFECT	MECHANISM OF INTERACTION
		(Phenobarbital) Phenobarbital toxicity may produced.	Phenobarbital and Phenytoin compate with Phenobarbital for the site of metabolism

Benzodiazepines: *Alprazolam, Chlordiazepoxide, Clonazepam, Clorazepate, Diazepam, Estazolam, Flurazepam, Halazepam, Lorazepam, Midazolam, Oxazepam, Quazepam, Temazepam, Triazolam*

DRUG	DRUG INTERACTION	EFFECT	MECHANISM OF INTERACTION
Benzodiazepines, Oxidative Metabolism-class [alprazolam, chlordiazepoxid, clonazepam, clorazepate, diazepam, estazolam, flurazepam, halazepam, midazolam, quazepam, triazolam]	Azole Antifungals [fluconazole, itraconazole, ketoconazole, miconazole, voriconazole]	Increased concentrations of benzodiazepine. Prolonged CNS depression and psychomotor impairment.	Azole Antifungals inhibit CYP3A4 mediated benzodiazepine metabolism. Azole Antifungals decrease reanal excretion of some benzodiazepine
	Clarithromycin	Increase serum concentration of Benzodiazepines Prolonged	inhibition of CYP3A4 by

DRUG	DRUG INTERACTION	EFFECT	MECHANISM OF INTERACTION
		sedation and respiratory depression.	Clarithromycin
	Diltiazem	Increased effects of benzodiazepine (diazepam, midazolam, triazolam). Prolonged sedation and respiratory depression.	Inhibition of CYP3A4 by diltiazem
	Ethanol	Additive CNS depressione with acute ethanol ingestion.	Additive CNS effects
	erythromycin	Increased concentrations of benzodiazepine. Prolonged sedation and respiratory depression.	inhibition of CYP3A4 by erythromycin
	Macrolide Antibiotics [clarithromycin, erythromycin, troleandomycin]	Increase serum concentration of Benzodiazepines Prolonged sedation and respiratory depression.	inhibition of CYP3A4 by Macrolide
	Protease Inhibitors	Increased concentrations of	Inhibition of CYP3A4 and p-

DRUG	DRUG INTERACTION	EFFECT	MECHANISM OF INTERACTION
	[indinavir, ritonavir, saquinavir]	benzodiazepine. Prolonged sedation and respiratory depression.	glycoprotein by indinavir that inhibit metabolism and transport of Benzodiazepines
	Ritonavir	Increased concentrations of benzodiazepine. Prolonged sedation and respiratory depression.	Inhibition of CYP3A4 and p-glycoprotein by indinavir that inhibit metabolism and transport of Benzodiazepines
	Theophylline derivatives	Diminish therapeuyic effect of benzodiazepines	Xanthine blockade of adenosine receptors oe xanthine induce metabolism of benzodiazepines

Buspirone

DRUG	DRUG INTERACTION	EFFECT	MECHANISM OF INTERACTION
Buspirone	Azole Antifungals [fluconazole, itraconazole, ketoconazole, miconazole, voriconazole]	Increased effects of buspirone.	CYP3A4 inhibition by Azole
	Macrolide Antibiotics [clarithromycin,	Increased effects of buspirone.	CYP3A4 inhibition by Macrolide

DRUG	DRUG INTERACTION	EFFECT	MECHANISM OF INTERACTION
	erythromycin, troleandomycin]		
	Rifamycins [rifabutin, rifampin]	Decreased effects of buspirone.	Induction of CYP3A4 isoenzyme by Rifamycins

Zolpidem

DRUG	DRUG INTERACTION	EFFECT	MECHANISM OF INTERACTION
Zolpidem	Ritonavir	Severe sedation and respiratory depression.	Inhibition of CYP3A4 and p-glycoprotein by indinavir that inhibit metabolism and transport of Zolpidem

ANTIPSYCHOTIC AGENTS

DRUG	DRUG INTERACTION	EFFECT	MECHANISM OF INTERACTION
Clozapine	Ritonavir	Increased concentrations of clozapine.	Inhibition of CYP3A4 and p-glycoprotein by ritonavir that mediate metabolism and transport of Clozapine
	Serotonin	Increased	SSRIs inhibit CYP

DRUG	DRUG INTERACTION	EFFECT	MECHANISM OF INTERACTION
	Reuptake Inhibitors [fluoxetine, fluvoxamine, sertraline]	concentrations of clozapine.	isoenzymes mediated Clozapine metabolism

Haloperidol

DRUG	DRUG INTERACTION	EFFECT	MECHANISM OF INTERACTION
Haloperidol	Azole Antifungals [fluconazole, itraconazole, ketoconazole]	Increased concentrations of haloperidol.	Inhibition of CYP3A4 mediated haloperidol metabolism by Azole
	Carbamazepine	Decreased effects of haloperidol.	Induction of CYP isoenzyme mediated haloperidol metabolism by carbamazepine
	Lithium	Alterations in consciousness, encephalopathy, extrapyramidal effects, fever, leukocytosis, and increased serum enzymes.	unknown
	Rifamycins [rifabutin, rifampin]	Decreased effects of haloperidol.	Induction of CYP3A4 by rifamycins

Phenothiazines: Acetophenazine, Chlorpromazine, Fluphenazine, Mesoridazine,Methotrimeprazine, Perphenazine, Prochlorperazine, Promazine,Promethazine, Propiomazine, Thiethylperazine, Thioridazine,Trifluoperazine, Triflupromazine

DRUG	DRUG INTERACTION	EFFECT	MECHANISM OF INTERACTION
Phenothiazines	Anticholinergics [atropine, belladonna, benztropine, biperiden, clidinium, dicyclomine, glycopyrrolate, hyoscyamine, isopropamide, mepenzolate, orphenadrine, oxybutynin, oxyphencyclimin, procyclidine, propantheline, scopolamine, trihexyphenidyl]	Excessive parasympatholytic effects may result in paralytic ileus, hyperthermia, heat stroke, and the anticholinergic intoxication syndrome.	Phenothiazines have anticholinergic properties
	Ethanol	Increased CNS depression and psychomotor impairment.	Additive CNS effects with acute ethanol ingestion
	fluoxetine	Increased risk of cardiac	Both drugs cause QTc—prolongation

DRUG	DRUG INTERACTION	EFFECT	MECHANISM OF INTERACTION
		arrhythmias, including torsades de pointes.	
	Paroxetine	Increased effects of phenothiazine. Increased risk of life-threatening cardiac arrhythmias with thioridazine.	Both drugs cause QTc—prolongation
chlorpromazine, thioridazine	fluconazole	Increase risk of ventricular fibrillation	Augmentation of QTc—prolongation by both drugs
	Propranolol,	Increased effects of one or both drugs.	Each drug inhibit the metabolism of other. Both drug produce hypotension and thus hypotension is augmented
	pindolol	Increased effects of one or both drugs.	Each drug inhibit the metabolism of other. Both drug produce

DRUG	DRUG INTERACTION	EFFECT	MECHANISM OF INTERACTION
			hypotension and thus hypotension is augmented
	Sparfloxacin	Increased risk of cardiac arrhythmias, including torsades de pointes.	Enhance the QTc-prolongatoion for each drug.

Chlorpromazine

DRUG	DRUG INTERACTION	EFFECT	MECHANISM OF INTERACTION
Chlorpromazine (See also Phenothiazines)	Meperidine	Excessive sedation and hypotension.	Increase renal excretion of normeperidine that have additive hypotensive and sedative effect

Thioridazine

DRUG	DRUG INTERACTION	EFFECT	MECHANISM OF INTERACTION
Thioridazine (See also Phenothiazines)	amiodarone	Enhance QTc—prolongation effect of amiodarone	Thioridazine and amiodarone both cause prolongation of QTc—interval
	Antiarrhythmic	Increased risk of	Thioridazine and

DRUG	DRUG INTERACTION	EFFECT	MECHANISM OF INTERACTION
	Agents [amiodarone, bretylium, disopyramide, procainamide, quinidine, sotalol]	cardiac arrhythmias, including torsades de pointes.	amiodarone both cause prolongation of QTc—interval
	Fluoxetine	Increased risk of cardiac arrhythmias, including torsades de pointes.	Both drugs cause QTc—prolongation
	Fluvoxamine	Increased risk of cardiac arrhythmias, including torsades de pointes.	Both drugs cause QTc—prolongation
	lidocaine	Increase serum concentration of thioridazine and enhance QTc intervals	Inhibition of CYP2D6 by lidocaine
	Pimozide	Increased risk of cardiac arrhythmias, including torsades de pointes.	Both drugs cause QTc—prolongation

PAIN MEDICATIONS

Non-Narcotic

Acetaminophen

DRUG	DRUG INTERACTION	EFFECT	MECHANISM OF INTERACTION
Acetaminophen	cholestyramine	Decrease serum concentration of acetaminophen	Decrease gastric absorption of acetaminophen
	Ethanol	Increased risk of acetaminophen-induced hepatotoxicity.	induction of hepatic microsomal enzymes during chronic alcohol use, which may result in accelerated metabolism of acetaminophen and increased production of potentially hepatotoxic metabolites
	Hydantoins [ethotoin, fosphenytoin, mephenytoin, phenytoin]	Increased risk of acetaminophen-induced hepatotoxicity.	Induction of CYP and UDPGTase isoenzyme mediated acetaminophen metabolism. Formation of acetaminophen metabolites which exceed glutathione binding capacity

DRUG	DRUG INTERACTION	EFFECT	MECHANISM OF INTERACTION
	Sulfinpyrazone	Increased risk of acetaminophen-induced hepatotoxicity.	Induction of acetaminophen metabolism (glucuronidation)
	Warfarin,	Increased effects of warfarin. (if acetaminophen is greater than 1.3 g/day continuously for greater than 1 week)	unknown

Aspirin

DRUG	DRUG INTERACTION	EFFECT	MECHANISM OF INTERACTION
Aspirin	Carbonic Anhydrase Inhibitors [acetazolamide, dichlorphenamid, methazolamide]	Increased risk of carbonic anhydrase inhibitor toxicity (CNS depression, metabolic acidosis). Salicylate toxicity also increased	Aspirin reduce protein binding of Carbonic Anhydrase Inhibitors and its renal clearance that increase acidity. Decrease in plasma PH can increase concentration of nonionized salicylate which more readily enter CNS

DRUG	DRUG INTERACTION	EFFECT	MECHANISM OF INTERACTION
	Corticosteroids [betamethasone, cortisone, desoxycorticoster one, dexamethasone, fludrocortisone, hydrocortisone, methylprednisolon paramethasone, prednisolone, prednisone, triamcinolone]	Decreased effects of salicylate. increase Corticosteroids adverse/ toxic effect (including GI tract ulceration and bleeding)	Induction of UDP-glucuronyl transferase activity. Both drugs have adverse gastric effect
	grisofulvin	Decrease therapeutic effects of salisylate	Decrease absorption of salisylate
	Heparin	Increased risk of bleeding.	Both drugs possess the potential to cause bleeding
	Insulin	Increased hypoglycemic effects of insulin.	Salicylates have blood lowering effect that add synergestic on insulin
	Ketorolac,	Increased risk of	Synergistic effect

DRUG	DRUG INTERACTION	EFFECT	MECHANISM OF INTERACTION
		ketorolac adverse effects(GI bleeding, renal dysfunction . . .)	
	Methotrexate,	Increased risk of methotrexate toxicity.	1.compate with methotrexate for excretion sites in the renal tubules 2. decrease renal excretion of methotrexate throughout renal prostaglandin senthesis inhibition
	Proton Pump Inhibitors [esomeprazole, lansoprazole, omeprazole, pantoprazole, rabeprazole]	decrease the oral bioavailability of aspirin and other salicylates.	acid suppression may reduce the lipophilic nature of aspirin, thereby adversely affecting its absorption from the gastrointestinal tract.
	Probenecid	Increased effects of salicylate	Competition on the renal excretion site
	Sulfonylureas	Increased hypoglycemic effects of sulfonylurea.	Salicylates have blood lowering effect that add synergestic on Sulfonylureas
	Valproic acid,	Increased free (unbound) concentrations of	Protein binding displacement

DRUG	DRUG INTERACTION	EFFECT	MECHANISM OF INTERACTION
		valproic acid.	
	Warfarin,	Increased effects of warfarin with large doses of salicylate. Increased risk of bleeding with any aspirin dose.	inhibit platelet aggregation

NARCOTIC

Alfentanil

DRUG	DRUG INTERACTION	EFFECT	MECHANISM OF INTERACTION
Alfentanil	Ethanol	additive CNS-depression and impairment of judgment, thinking, and psychomotor skills.	additive CNS-effects
	Clarithromycin	Increase serum concentration of alfentanil	inhibition of CYP3A4 by Clarithromycin
	erythromycin	Increase serum concentration of alfentanil	inhibition of CYP3A4 by erythromycin

Codeine

DRUG	DRUG INTERACTION	EFFECT	MECHANISM OF INTERACTION
Codeine	Quinidine	Decreased effects of codeine.	Inhibition of CYP2D6 mediated codeine metabolism by quinidine

Fentanyl

DRUG	DRUG INTERACTION	EFFECT	MECHANISM OF INTERACTION
Fentanyl	Amiodarone,	Increase concentration of Fentanyl. Increased risk of profoundbradycardia sinus arrest and hypotension	Inhibition of CYP3A4 mediated Fentanyl metabolism by amiodarone
	Tetracycline	Increase serum concentration of fentanyl	Tetracycline is moderate CYP3A4 inhibitor

Meperidine

DRUG	DRUG INTERACTION	EFFECT	MECHANISM OF INTERACTION
Meperidine	MAO Inhibitors [isocarboxazid, phenelzine,	Agitation, seizures, diaphoresis and fever. May	Additive effect on serotonin, Meperidine block

DRUG	DRUG INTERACTION	EFFECT	MECHANISM OF INTERACTION
	selegiline, tranylcypromine]	progress to coma, apnea, and death.	its reuptake and MAOI reduc its metabolism
	Phenothiazines [chlorpromazine]	Excessive sedation and hypotension.	Increase renal excretion of normeperidine that have additive hypotensive and sedative effect
	Ritonavir	Decreased efficacy of meperidine and increased risk of neurologic toxicity.	induction of CYP2B6, CYP2C19 that metabolite Meperidine to highly toxic normeperidine
	Sibutramine	Increased risk of serotonin syndrome (CNS irritability, shivering, myoclonus, altered consciousness).	Meperidine Increase serotonin activity, Sibutramine inhibit serotonin reuptake

Methadone

DRUG	DRUG INTERACTION	EFFECT	MECHANISM OF INTERACTION
Methadone	Barbiturates [amobarbital, aprobarbital, butabarbital, butalbital,	Decreased effects of methadone. Possible with— drawal symptoms in patients on	Induction of metabolic enzymes mediated Methadone metabolism

214

Qutaiba A. Ibrahim

mephobarbital, pentobarbital, phenobarbital, primidone]	chronic methadone therapy.	
Fluvoxamine	Increased concentrations of methadone.	Fluvoxamine inhibit CYP2C9, CYP2D6, CYP3A4 mediated Methadone metabolism
Hydantoins [ethotoin, fosphenytoin, mephenytoin, phenytoin]	Decreased effects of methadone. Possible with-drawal symptoms in patientson chronic methadone therapy.	Induction of hepat metabolism of methadone by Hydantoins
Rifampin	Decreased effectsof methadone. Possible with-drawal symptoms in patientson chronic methadone therapy.	Induction of CYP2B6, CYP2C9, CYP3A4 mediated methadone metabolism by rifampin

Morphine

DRUG	DRUG INTERACTION	EFFECT	MECHANISM OF INTERACTION
Morphine	Rifamycins [rifabutin, rifampin, rifapentine]	Decreased analgesic effectsof morphine.	Induction of CYP3A4 and CYP2C8 by rifampin

Propoxyphene

DRUG	DRUG INTERACTION	EFFECT	MECHANISM OF INTERACTION
Propoxyphene	Carbamazepine,	Increased concentration and CNS depressant effect of carbamazepine.	Inhibition of CYP3A4 by Propoxyphene. Synergestic CNS depressant effect of both drugs
	Ritonavir	Increased risk of propoxyphene toxicity (seizures, respiratorydepression, apnea, cardiac arrhythmias, pulmonary edema).	CYP3A4 inhibition by ritonavir

HYPOGLYCEMIC AGENTS

Insulin

DRUG	DRUG INTERACTION	EFFECT	MECHANISM OF INTERACTION
Insulin	ACEIs	Enhance hypoglycemic effect of insulin	ACEI have various effect both islet structure and function as well as enhancing insulin sensitivity
	Beta-Blockers, Noncardio—	Prolonged hypoglycemia with	Blocking of beta receptors in

DRUG	DRUG INTERACTION	EFFECT	MECHANISM OF INTERACTION
	Selective [carteolol, nadolol, penbutolol, pindolol, propranolol, timolol]	masking of hypoglycemic signs/symptoms (tachycardia)	pancrease that regulate insulin release, and inhibition of tackycardia mediated by Epinephrine
	Ethanol	Increased hypoglycemic effects of insulin.	Ethanol cause inhibition of gluconeogenesis as well as the counterregulatory response to hypoglycemia
	MAO Inhibitors [isocarboxazid, phenelzine, tranylcypromine]	Increased hypoglycemic effects of insulin.	stimulating insulin secretion
	Salicylates [aspirin, bismuth subsalicylate, choline salicylate, magnesium salicylate, salsalate, sodium salicylate, sodium thiosalicylate]	Increased hypoglycemic effects of insulin.	Salicylates have blood lowering effect that add synergestic on insulin
	quinolone	Hypoglycemia 1-2 days of initiating quinolone therapy. Hypoglycemia tend to occur later in therapy lend	Insulin may simply enhance the insulin-secreting effect of quinolone

ORAL HYPOGLYCEMIC AGENTS

Metformin

DRUG	DRUG INTERACTION	EFFECT	MECHANISM OF INTERACTION
Metformin	cephalexin	Cephalexin may increase serum concentration of metformin	Impaired renal clearance of metformin by cephalexin (competitive inhibitors)
	Cimetidine	Increased concentrations of metformin.	Inhibition of OCTs resulting in reduction in metformin renal tubular secretion, in addition to inhibition of human multidrug and toxin extrusion1 (hMATE1/SLC47A1) and hMATE2-K (SLC47A2) mediated metformin transport
	Iodinated Contrast Materials, IV	Increased risk of lactic acidosis.	Both agents cause reduction in renal function that result in lactic acidosis
	Thiazide Diuretics [bendroflumethia zide, benzthiazide,	Decrease the therapeutic effect of metformin	Hypokalemia induced by thiazide diuretics cause decrease in the effect of metformin

DRUG	DRUG INTERACTION	EFFECT	MECHANISM OF INTERACTION
	chlorothiazide, chlorthalidone, hydrochlorothiazide, hydroflumethiazide indapamide, methyclothiazide, metolazone, polythiazide, quinethazone, trichlormethiazide		

Sulfonylureas:

Acetohexamide, Chlorpropamide, Glimepride, Glipizide, Glyburide, Tolazamide, Tolbutamide

DRUG	DRUG INTERACTION	EFFECT	MECHANISM OF INTERACTION
Sulfonylureas	ACEI	Enhance hypoglycemic effect of sulphonylureas	ACEI have various effect both islet structure and function as well ason the physiologic response to hypoglycemia

DRUG	DRUG INTERACTION	EFFECT	MECHANISM OF INTERACTION
	Azole Antifungals [fluconazole, itraconazole, ketoconazole]	Increased hypoglycemic effects of Sulfonylureas	Inhibition of CYP2C9 isoenzymes by azole antifungal
	Chloramphenicol	Increased hypoglycemic effects of sulfonylurea.	Unclear, possibly due to inhibition of sulfonylurea metabolism
	Diazoxide	Decreased hypoglycemic effects of sulfonylurea.	Diazoxide interfere with blood glucose control because they can cause hyperglycemia, glucose intolerance, new-onset diabetes mellitus, and/or exacerbation of preexisting diabetes.
	Ethanol,	Prolonged hypoglycemia. Disulfiram-like reaction when taken with chlorpropamide.	inhibition of gluconeogenesis and inhibition of the counterregulatory response to hypoglycemia.
	MAO Inhibitors [isocarboxazid, phenelzine, tranylcypromine]	Increased hypoglycemic effects of sulfonylurea.	MAO Inhibitors increase the risk of hypoglycemia by enhancing insulin sensitivity

DRUG	DRUG INTERACTION	EFFECT	MECHANISM OF INTERACTION
	Phenylbutazones [oxyphenbutazone, phenylbutazone]	Increased hypoglycemic effects of sulfonylurea.	Phenylbutazones stimulating insulin secretion
	Rifamycins [rifabutin, rifampin, rifapentine]	Decreased concentrations of sulfonylurea.	Induction of CYP2C9 by rifamycins
	Salicylates [aspirin, choline salicylate, magnesium salicylate, salsalate, sodium salicylate, sodium thiosalicylate]	Increased hypoglycemic effects of sulfonylurea.	Salicylates have blood lowering effect that add synergestic on Sulfonylureas
	Sulfonamides [sulfacytine, sulfadiazine, sulfamethizole, sulfamethoxazole, sulfasalazine, sulfisoxazole, multiple sulfonamides]	Enhance the hypoglycemic effect of sulfonylurea. Exception: Glyburide	Inhibition of Sulfonylureas metabolism by sulfonamides. Displacement of Sulfonylureas from plasma protein binding site
	Thiazide Diuretics [bendroflumethiazide, benzthiazide, chlorothiazide, chlorthalidone, hydrochlorothiazid	Increased fasting blood glucose. Decreased hypoglycemic effects of sulfonylurea.	Thiazide impair insulin sensitivity, increase insulin resistance, increase basal plasma glucose concentration.

DRUG	DRUG INTERACTION	EFFECT	MECHANISM OF INTERACTION
	hydroflumethiazide indapamide, methyclothiazide, metolazone, quinethazone, trichlormethiazide		All of thes may result from hypokalemia produced by Thiazide
	Quinolones [gatifloxacin, moxifloxacin, sparfloxacin]	Quinolones may enhance the hypoglycemic effect of sulfonylureas(early in the course of administration) Quinolones may diminish the hypoglycemic effect of sulfonylureas in long-term combination	Quinolones have dual effects on pancreatic islet cell, initially stimulate insulin release ,but inhibiting insulin release after long—term

Chlorpropamide

DRUG	DRUG INTERACTION	EFFECT	MECHANISM OF INTERACTION
Chlorpropamide *(See also sulfonylureas)*	Allopurinol	Increase serum concentration of Chlorpropamide	Competition for renal excretion
	Ammonium chloride	Increase serum concentration of Chlorpropamide	Acidity of urine is increased by ammonium chloride that cause Chlorpropamide to be in unionized form that more readily absorbed
	Dicumarol	Increased hypoglycemic effects of chlorpropamide.	possibly by inhibiting Dicumarol hepatic metabolism.
	Ethanol	disulfiram-like reaction (flushing, headache, and nausea)	inhibits aldehyde dehydrogenase
	Urinary Alkalinizers [potassium citrate, sodium acetate, sodium bicarbonate, sodium citrate, sodium lactate, tromethamine]	Decrease therapeutic effect of chlorpropamide	Increased renal elimination of chlorpropamide.

Glimepride

DRUG	DRUG INTERACTION	EFFECT	MECHANISM OF INTERACTION
Glimepride *(See also* sulfonylureas*)*	Fluconazole	Increased hypoglycemic effects of Glimepride.	Inhibition of CYP2C9 mediated Glimepride metabolism by Fluconazole

Tolbutamide

DRUG	DRUG INTERACTION	EFFECT	MECHANISM OF INTERACTION
Tolbutamide *(See also* sulfonylureas*)*	Aprepitant	Decrease serum concentration of tolbutamide	Aprepitant-mediated induction of CYP2C9 which mediated metabolism of tolbutamide
	Dicumarol	Increased hypoglycemic effects of tolbutamide.	possibly by inhibiting Dicumarol hepatic metabolism.
	Fluconazole	Increased hypoglycemic effects of tolbutamide.	Inhibition of CYP2C9 mediated tolbutamide metabolism by Fluconazole
	Sulfinpyrazone	Increased hypoglycemic effects of	Inhibition of CYP2C9 mediated tolbutamide

DRUG	DRUG INTERACTION	EFFECT	MECHANISM OF INTERACTION
		tolbutamide.	metabolism by Sulfinpyrazone

HYPOLIPIDEMIC AGENTS

Cholestyramine

DRUG	DRUG INTERACTION	EFFECT	MECHANISM OF INTERACTION
Cholestyramine	acetaminophen	Decrease serum concentration of acetaminophen	Decrease gastric absorption of acetaminophen
	amiodarone	Decrease effect of amiodarone	Binding of amiodarone and Cholestyramine in GIT that inhibit its absorption
	Digoxin,	Decreased concentrations of digoxin.	Cholestyramine bind digoxin in the GI tract, that inhibit digoxin absorption
	HMG-CoA Reductase Inhibitors	Decreased GI absorption of HMG-CoA reductase inhibitor.	Cholestyramine bind HMG-CoA Reductase Inhibitors in GIT that reduce its absorption
	Hydrocortisone,	Decreased GI absorption of hydrocortisone.	Cholestyramine bind Hydrocortisone in GIT that reduce its absorption

DRUG	DRUG INTERACTION	EFFECT	MECHANISM OF INTERACTION
	Furosemide,	Decreased GIT absorption of furosemide.	Cholestyramine bind furosemide in GIT that reduce its absorption
	Levothyroxine,	Decreased GI absorption of levothyroxine.	Cholestyramine bind Levothyroxine in GIT that reduce its absorption
	tetracycline	Decrease absorption of tetracycline	Colestipol bind to tetracycline in GIT. The mechanism of other bile acid sequestrant is unknown
	Valproic Acid	Decreased therapeutic effect of valproic acid.	Cholestyramine may interfere with the gastrointestinal absorption of valproic acid reducing serum concentrations, bioavailability and therapeutic effect
	Warfarin,	Decreased effects of warfarin.	Cholestyramine bind warfarin in the GI tract both upon initial presentation and during the course of enterohepatic cycle

Clofibrate

DRUG	DRUG INTERACTION	EFFECT	MECHANISM OF INTERACTION
Clofibrate	hydrocortisone	Decreased GI absorption of hydrocortisone.	Clofibrate bind Hydrocortisone in GIT that reduce its absorption
	Warfarin,	Increased effects of warfarin.	1.Fibric Acids cause displacement of warfarin from protein binding sites. 2.Increase affinity of of anticoagulant for binding sites 3. fenofibrate is inhibitor for CYP2C9

Colestipol

DRUG	DRUG INTERACTION	EFFECT	MECHANISM OF INTERACTION
Colestipol	HMG-CoA Reductase Inhibitors	Decreased GI absorption of HMG-CoA reductase inhibitor.	Colestipol bind HMG-CoA Reductase Inhibitors in GIT that reduce its absorption
	Hydrocortisone	Decreased GI	Colestipol bind

DRUG	DRUG INTERACTION	EFFECT	MECHANISM OF INTERACTION
		absorption of hydrocortisone.	hydrocortisone in GIT that reduce its absorption
	Loop Diuretics	Decreased GI absorption of furosemide.	Colestipol bind furosemide in GIT that reduce its absorption

Gemfibrozil

DRUG	DRUG INTERACTION	EFFECT	MECHANISM OF INTERACTION
Gemfibrozil	HMG-CoA Reductase Inhibitors	Increased risk of severe myopathy and rhabdomyolysis.	Gemfibrozil inhibit CYP2C8 and OATP1B1 mediated metabolism and transport of HMG-CoA Reductase Inhibitors. In addition Gemfibrozil associated by rhabdomyolysis and other muscular toxicity and myopathy

Probucol

DRUG	DRUG INTERACTION	EFFECT	MECHANISM OF INTERACTION
Probucol	Cyclosporine,	Decreased concentrations of cyclosporine.	Decrease in gastric absorption of cyclosporine by Probucol

HMG-CoA Reductase

Atorvastatin, Fluvastatin, Lovastatin, Pravastatin, Rosuvastatin, Simvastatin

DRUG	DRUG INTERACTION	EFFECT	MECHANISM OF INTERACTION
HMG-CoA Reductase Inhibitors	Azole Antifungals [fluconazole, itraconazole, ketoconazole, miconazole, voriconazole]	Increased risk of rhabdomyolysis.	Azole Antifungals inhibit CYP2C9 and CYP3A4 mediated HMG-CoA Reductase Inhibitors metabolism
	Bile Acid Sequestrants [cholestyramine, colestipol]	Decreased GI absorption of HMG-CoA reductase inhibitor.	Bile Acid Sequestrants bind HMG-CoA Reductase Inhibitors in GIT that reduce its absorption
	amiodarone	Enhance risk of severe myopathy and rhabdomyolysis	Amiodarone decrease metabolism of HMG-CoA

DRUG	DRUG INTERACTION	EFFECT	MECHANISM OF INTERACTION
			Reductase Inhibitors by by CYP3A4 inhibition
	Cyclosporine	Increased risk of rhabdomyolysis.	Inhibition of CYP3A4 mediated HMG-CoA Reductase Inhibitors metabolism by Cyclosporine
	Diltiazem	Increased risk of rhabdomyolysis. [Exceptions: fluvastatin, pravastatin]	Inhibition of CYP3A4-mediated HMG-CoA Reductase Inhibitors metabolism by diltiazem
	Gemfibrozil	Increased risk of severe myopathy and rhabdomyolysis.	Gemfibrozil inhibit CYP2C8 and OATP1B1 mediated metabolism and transport of HMG-CoA Reductase Inhibitors. In addition Gemfibrozil associated by rhabdomyolysis and other muscular toxicity and myopathy
	Macrolide Antibiotics [azithromycin,	Increased risk of severemyopathy and	Inhibition of CYP3A4 mediated metabolism

DRUG	DRUG INTERACTION	EFFECT	MECHANISM OF INTERACTION
	clarithromycin, erythromycin]	rhabdomyolysis. [Exceptions: fluvastatin, pravastatin]	(simvastatin, lovastatin, atorvastatin)
	Nefazodone	Increased risk of rhabdomyolysis. [Exceptions: fluvastatin, pravastatin]	Inhibition of CYP2D6 mediated HMG-CoA Reductase Inhibitors metabolism by Nefazodone
	Proton Pump Inhibitors [esomeprazole, lansoprazole, omeprazole, pantoprazole, rabeprazole]	increase the plasma concentrations of atorvastatin and the associated risk of myopathy.	competitive inhibition of intestinal P-glycoprotein, resulting in decreased drug secretion into the intestinal lumen and increased drug bioavailability. Another, perhaps minor mechanism is competitive inhibition of CYP450 3A4 metabolism.
	Rifamycins [rifabutin, rifampin, rifapentine]	Decreased effects of statin. [Exception: pravastatin]	Induction of CYP3A4 by rifamycins
	Verapamil	Increased risk of rhabdomyolysis. [Exceptions: fluvastatin,	Inhibition of CYP3A4-mediated HMG-CoA Reductase

DRUG	DRUG INTERACTION	EFFECT	MECHANISM OF INTERACTION
		pravastatin]	Inhibitors metabolism by verapamil
	warfarin	Increased effects of warfarin.	Inhibition of CYP2C9 isoenzymes mediated warfarin metabolism

Lovastatin

DRUG	DRUG INTERACTION	EFFECT	MECHANISM OF INTERACTION
Lovastatin (See also HMG-CoA Reductase Inhibitors)	Cyclosporine	Increased risk of rhabdomyolysis.	Inhibition of CYP3A4 mediated Lovastatin metabolism by Cyclosporine

GASTROINTESTINAL AGENTS

Histamine H2-Antagonists Cimetidine, Famotidine, Nizatidine, Ranitidine

DRUG	DRUG INTERACTION	EFFECT	MECHANISM OF INTERACTION
Histamine H2-Antagonists	Ketoconazole,	Decreased GI absorption of ketoconazole.	Ketoconazole required acidic media for dissolution, Histamine H2-Antagonists

DRUG	DRUG INTERACTION	EFFECT	MECHANISM OF INTERACTION
			decrease the rate of absorption of Ketoconazole

Cimetidine

DRUG	DRUG INTERACTION	EFFECT	MECHANISM OF INTERACTION
Cimetidine*(See also* Histamine H2-Antagonists*)*	Acyclovir	increase serum concentration of acyclovir	Competition of the drugs for the renal tubule secretion sites
	Beta-Blockers	Increased concentrations of beta-blocker.	inhibition of metabolism that is not excreted unchanged in urine
	Calcium channel blockers	Increase bioavailability of Calcium channel blockers	Inhibition of CYP3A4 by cimetidine
	Carbamazepine,	Increased concentrations of carbamazepine.	Cimetidine inhibit metabolism of carbamazepine and/or effect its absorption
	Lidocaine,	Increased concentrations of lidocaine.	inhibition of hepatic CYP450 metabolism and reduced hepatic blood flow

DRUG	DRUG INTERACTION	EFFECT	MECHANISM OF INTERACTION
	Metformin,	Increased concentrations of metformin.	Inhibition of OCTs resulting in reduction in metformin renal tubular secretion, in addition to inhibition of human multidrug and toxin extrusion1 (hMATE1/SLC47A1) and hMATE2-K (SLC47A2) mediated metformin transport
	Moricizine	Increased concentrations of moricizine. increase the risk of ECG changes	cimetidine may inhibit the hepatic metabolism of moricizine. Bioavailability
	Nifedipine,	Increased effects of nifedipine.	Inhibition of CYP3A4 by cimetidine
	Hydantoins [ethotoin, fosphenytoin, mephenytoin, phenytoin],	Increased concentrations of Hydantoins.	Inhibition of CYP isoenzyme mediated
	Praziquantel	Increased concentrations of praziquantel.	Inhibition of CYP3A4 mediated Praziquantel metabolism by cimetidine

DRUG	DRUG INTERACTION	EFFECT	MECHANISM OF INTERACTION
	Procainamide,	Increased concentrationsof procainamide and N-acetylprocainamide	Cimetidine decrease renal excretion of procainamide
	Quinidine,	Increased concentrations of quinidine.	Inhibition of CYP3A4 mediated Quinidine metabolism by quinidine
	Serotonin Reuptake Inhibitor paroxetine, sertraline]	Increase serum concentration of SSRIs	CYP3A4 inhibition by cimetidine
	Theophylline,	Increased concentrations of theophylline.	Inhibition of CYP isoenzyme mediated theophylline metabolism
	Tricyclic Antidepressants	Increased concentrations of tricyclic antidepressant.	Inhibition of CYP2C19 mediated tricyclic antidepressant metabolism by Cimetidine
	Warfarin,	Increased effects of warfarin.	Cimetidine inhibit hepatic metabolism of warfarin (hydroxylation)

Phosphate Binders/Antacids

Aluminum Salts (Aluminum Carbonate, Aluminum Hydroxide) Calcium Salts (Calcium Carbonate, Calcium Acetate), Magnesium Salts (Magnesium Carbonate, Magnesium Hydroxide)

DRUG	DRUG INTERACTION	EFFECT	MECHANISM OF INTERACTION
Phosphate Binders/ Antacids-class	cephalosporins	Decrease absorption of cephalosporins	formation of Chelate between cephalosporins and antiacids
	Iron Salts (Oral) [ferrous fumarate, ferrous gluconate, ferrous sulfate,iron polysaccharide]	Decreased GI absorption of iron.	Formation of less foluble iron complexes
	Ketoconazole,	Decrease concentration of Ketoconazole	Ketoconazole tablets dissolved in acidic media, Antacids decrease Ketoconazole dissolution that decrease its absorption
	Quinidine,	Increased concentrations/ toxic effect of of quinidine.	Quinidine renal excretion decreased in alkaline urine produced by antacids
	Quinolone	Decreased GI	The carbonyl and

DRUG	DRUG INTERACTION	EFFECT	MECHANISM OF INTERACTION
	antibiotics	absorption of quinolone.	4-oxo functional groups on the antibiotics forms a chelate with cations of the antiacid
	Sodium Polystyrene Sulfonate (Kayexalate),	Increased risk of metabolic alkalosis. Decreased potassium binding effects of resin.	Sodium Polystyrene Sulfonate binds magnesium and calcium ion and thereby prevent binding and neutralizing of bicarbonate ion in small intestine
	Tetracyclines,	Decreased GI absorption of tetracycline.	formation of Chelate between tetracycline and antiacids

Calcium Carbonate

DRUG	DRUG INTERACTION	EFFECT	MECHANISM OF INTERACTION
Calcium Carbonate

(See also Phosphate Binders/ Antacids-class) | Verapamil, | Reverse clinical effects and toxicities of verapamil. | Calcium-containing products may decrease the effectiveness of calcium channel blockers by saturating calcium channels with calcium. |

Calcium Acetate

DRUG	DRUG INTERACTION	EFFECT	MECHANISM OF INTERACTION
Calcium Acetate (See also Phosphate Binders/ Antacids-class)	Verapamil,	Reverse clinical effects and toxicities of verapamil.	Calcium-containing products may decrease the effectiveness of calcium channel blockers by saturating calcium channels with calcium.

Sevelamer

DRUG	DRUG INTERACTION	EFFECT
Sevelamer	No drug-drug interaction studies were performed in humans. There is a possibility that sevelamer hydrochloride may bind concomitantly administered drugs and decrease their bioavailability.	

Proton Pump Inhibitors (PPIs)

Esomeprazole, Lansoprazole, Omeprazole, Pantoprazole, Rabeprazole

DRUG	DRUG INTERACTION	EFFECT	MECHANISM OF INTERACTION
Proton Pump Inhibitors-class	Azole Antifungals[fluconazole, itraconazole,	Decrease serum concentration of Azole antifungals.	Decreased GI absorption of Azole antifungals.

DRUG	DRUG INTERACTION	EFFECT	MECHANISM OF INTERACTION
	ketoconazole]		
		Increase serum concentration of Proton Pump Inhibitors	Ketoconazole inhibit CYP3A4 mediated Proton Pump Inhibitors metabolism,
	aspirin	decrease the oral bioavailability of aspirin and other salicylates.	acid suppression may reduce the lipophilic nature of aspirin, thereby adversely affecting its absorption from the GIT.
	HMG-CoA Reductase Inhibitors (Atorvastatin Fluvastatin Lovastatin Pravastatin Rosuvastatin Simvastatin)	increase the plasma concentrations of atorvastatin and the associated risk of myopathy.	competitive inhibition of intestinal P-glycoprotein, resulting in decreased drug secretion into the intestinal lumen and increased drug bioavailability. Another, perhaps minor mechanism is competitive inhibition of CYP450 3A4 metabolism.
	Iron Salts (Oral) [ferrous fumarate, ferrous gluconate, ferrous sulfate, iron	Decrease serum concentration of iron	Increase in gastrointestinal PH associated with decrease in iron absorption. Also stomach acidity

DRUG	DRUG INTERACTION	EFFECT	MECHANISM OF INTERACTION
	polysaccharide]		required for releasing iron from dietary sources
	Vitamin B12 (cyanocobalamin)	Decrease Vitamin B12 effect	interfere with the gastrointestinal absorption of vitamin B12, a process that is dependent on the presence of gastric acid and pepsin
	clopidogrel	Coadministration with proton pump inhibitors (PPIs) may reduce the cardioprotective effects of clopidogrel.	The proposed mechanism is PPI inhibition of the CYP450 2C19-mediated metabolic bioactivation of clopidogrel

Miscellaneous Gastrointestinal Agents

Metoclopramide

DRUG	DRUG INTERACTION	EFFECT	MECHANISM OF INTERACTION
Metoclopramide	Cyclosporine,	Increased concentrations of cyclosporine.	The prokinetic effect of metoclopramide on GI tract, which result in more rapid transport of cyclosporine

DRUG	DRUG INTERACTION	EFFECT	MECHANISM OF INTERACTION
	Digoxin,	Decreased concentrations of digoxin.	metoclopramide-induced stimulation of gastric motility, which may decrease digoxin absorption..
	levodopa	Decrease therapeutic effect of levodopa	Antidopaminergic effect of metoclopramide decrease the effect of dopamine agonist

Sodium Polystyrene Sulfonate (Kayexalate)

DRUG	DRUG INTERACTION	EFFECT	MECHANISM OF INTERACTION
Sodium PolystyreneSulfonate (Kayexalate)	Phosphate Binders/ Antacids [aluminum-magnesium hydroxide, calcium carbonate]	Increased risk of metabolic alkalosis. Decreased potassium binding effects of resin.	Sodium Polystyrene Sulfonate binds magnesium and calcium ion and thereby prevent binding and neutralizing of bicarbonate ion in small intestine

Sucralfate

DRUG	DRUG INTERACTION	EFFECT	MECHANISM OF INTERACTION
Sucralfate	digoxin	Decrease effect of digoxin	Binding of both drug in the GIT and thereby decrease absorption of digoxin
	levothyroxine	Decreased GI absorption of levothyroxine.	Formation of poorly absorbed complex
	Quinolones [gatifloxacin, moxifloxacin, sparfloxacin],	Decreased GI absorption of quinolone.	Formation of insoluble complex between aluminium of sucralfate and quinolone
	phenytoin	reduce phenytoin therapeutic effect	Sucralfate may interfere with the absorption of oral phenytoin
	quinidine	Decreased GI absorption of quinidine	Binding of both drug in the GIT and thereby decrease absorption of quinidine
	tetracyclines	Decrease serum concentration of tetracyclines	Binding of both drug in the GIT and thereby decrease absorption of tetracyclines

CORTICOSTEROIDS

Betamethasone, Corticotropin, Cortisone, Cosyntropin,
Dexamethasone, Fludrocortisone, Hydrocortisone,
Methylprednisolone, Prednisolone, Prednisone,
Triamcinolone

DRUG	DRUG INTERACTION	EFFECT	MECHANISM OF INTERACTION
Corticosteroids-class	Anticholinesterases [ambenonium, edrophonium, neostigmine, pyridostigmine]	Corticosteroids antagonize effect of anticholinesterases in myasthenia gravis.	Corticosteroids capable of causing an exacerbation of muscle weakness in myasthenia gravis
	Aspirin,	Decreased effects of salicylate. increase Corticosteroids adverse/ toxic effect (including GI tract ulceration and bleeding)	Induction of UDP-glucuronyl transferase activity. Both drugs have adverse gastric effect
	Barbiturates [amobarbital, aprobarbital, butabarbital, butalbital, mephobarbital, pentobarbital, phenobarbital, primidone]	Decreased effects of corticosteroid.	Induction of CYP isoenzyme mediated Corticosteroids metabolism by Corticosteroids
	Estrogens [chlorotrianisen,	Increased effects of Corticosteroids.	1.change in Corticosteroids

DRUG	DRUG INTERACTION	EFFECT	MECHANISM OF INTERACTION
	conjugated estrogens, diethylstilbesterol, esterified estrogens, estradiol, estrone, estropipate, ethinyl estradiol, quinestrol]		metabolism 2.change in the ability of Corticosteroids to pined to proteins
	Macrolide antibiotics (clarithromycin, erythromycin, telithromycin	Increase therapeutic/ toxoic effect of corticosteroides	inhibition of CYP3A4 by erythromycin
	Hydantoins [ethotoin, fosphenytoin, mephenytoin, phenytoin]	Decreased effects of corticosteroid.	induce the CYP450 3A4 hepatic metabolism of corticosteroids and increase their clearance and decrease their half-lives
	Rifamycins [rifabutin, rifampin, rifapentine]	Decreased effects of corticosteroid.	Induction of CYP isoenzymes by rifamycins

Dexamethasone

DRUG	DRUG INTERACTION	EFFECT	MECHANISM OF INTERACTION
Dexamethasone *(See also Corticosteroids-class)*	Azole Antifungals [fluconazole, itraconazole, ketoconazole]	Increased effects of dexamethasone.	Inhibition of CYP3A4 by Azole Antifungals

Hydrocortisone

DRUG	DRUG INTERACTION	EFFECT	MECHANISM OF INTERACTION
Hydrocortisone *(See also Corticosteroids-class)*	Azole Antifungals [fluconazole, itraconazole, ketoconazole]	Increased effects of hydrocortisone.	Inhibition of CYP3A4 by Azole Antifungals
	Bile Acid Sequestrants [cholestyramine, colestipol]	Decreased GI absorption of hydrocortisone.	Cholestyramine bind Hydrocortisone in GIT that reduce its absorption

Methylprednisolone

DRUG	DRUG INTERACTION	EFFECT	MECHANISM OF INTERACTION
Methylprednisolone	Azole Antifungals [fluconazole,	Increased effects of	Inhibition of CYP3A4 by Azole

	itraconazole, ketoconazole]	methylprednisolon e.	Antifungals
(See also Corticosteroids-class)			

Prednisolone and Prednisone

DRUG	DRUG INTERACTION	EFFECT	MECHANISM OF INTERACTION
Prednisolone and Prednisone (See also Corticosteroids)	Azole Antifungals [fluconazole, itraconazole, ketoconazole]	Increased effects of corticosteroid.	Inhibition of CYP3A4 by Azole Antifungals

VITAMINS

Folic acid

DRUG	DRUG INTERACTION	EFFECT	MECHANISM OF INTERACTION
Folic acid	phenobarbital	Decrease serum concentration of Phenobarbital	Inhibition of parahydroxylation of Phenobarbital by folic acid
	Phenytoin,	Decreased concentrations of phenytoin.	Folic acid is a cofactor for phenytoin metabolism thus high Folic acid can increase in affinity of phenytoin to metabolizing enzymes

Vitamin E (Tocopherol)

DRUG	DRUG INTERACTION	EFFECT	MECHANISM OF INTERACTION
Vitamin E (Tocopherol)	orlistate	Decrease serum concentration of vitamins(fat soluble)	Inhibition of gastric and pancreatic lipase
	Warfarin,	Increased effects of warfarin.	Vitamin E interfere with vitamin K— dependant process of clotting factors production

Vitamin K (Phytonadione)

DRUG	DRUG INTERACTION	EFFECT	MECHANISM OF INTERACTION
Vitamin K (Phytonadione) (food sourse)	orlistate	Decrease serum concentration of vitamins(fat soluble)	Inhibition of gastric and pancreatic lipase
	Warfarin,	Decreased or reversed effects of warfarin.	Vitamin K interfere with ability of warfarin to inhibit production of clotting factors

TRANSPLANT IMMUNOSUPPRESSANTS

Cyclosporine

DRUG	DRUG INTERACTION	EFFECT	MECHANISM OF INTERACTION
Cyclosporine	Amiodarone	Increased concentrations/ toxicity of cyclosporine.	Inhibition of cyclosporine metabolism by amiodarone
	ACEI	Increase risk of cyclosporine nephrotoxicity	Cyclosporine cause renal afferent vessel constriction, increasing the kidney reliance on angiotensin II to maintain adequate perfusion. ACEI decrease angiotensin II concentration
	Androgens [danazol, methyltestosterone]	Nandrolone enhance the hepatotoxic effect of cyclosporine by increasing plasma concentration of cyclosporine	Unknwn, thought to be due to inhibition of hepatic metabolism of cyclosporine
	Azole Antifungals [fluconazole, itraconazole, ketoconazole]	Increased concentrations of cyclosporine.	Inhibtion of CYP3A4 mediated cyclosporine metabolism by Azole Antifungals. Also inhibition of p-glycoprotein that

DRUG	DRUG INTERACTION	EFFECT	MECHANISM OF INTERACTION
			interfere with cyclosporine transport
	Probucol	Decreased concentrations of cyclosporine.	Decrease in gastric absorption of cyclosporine by Probucol
	Carbamazepine	Decreased concentrations of cyclosporine.	Induction of CYP3A4 mediated Cyclosporine metabolism by carbamazepine
	Calcium channel blockers (amlodipine, diltiazem,isradipine felodipine, nicardipine, nifedipine, verapamil)	Increased concentrations of Calcium channel blockers.	Inhibition of CYP3A4 by Cyclosporine decrease Calcium channel blockers metabolism
	Carvedilol	Increased concentrations of cyclosporine.	Carvedolol mediated inhibition of p-glycoprotein that effect transport of cyclosporine
	Colchicine	Increased risk of cyclosporine toxicity (GI, hepatic, renal, neuromuscular).	competitive inhibition of P-glycoprotein (P-gp) efflux transporter in the intestine,

DRUG	DRUG INTERACTION	EFFECT	MECHANISM OF INTERACTION
			renal proximal tubule and liver, resulting in increased drug absorption and decreased excretion
	Digoxin,	Increased concentrations of digoxin.	Cyclosporine inhibit p-glycoprotein activity that decrease the presentation of digoxin to the metabolic enzymes
	Etoposide	Increased concentrations/ toxicity of etoposide.	Inhibition of CYP3A4 mediated Etoposide mertabolism and p-glycoprotein mediated Etoposide transport
	Foscarnet,	Increased risk of renal failure.	synergistic nephrotoxicity
	Hydantoins [ethotoin, fosphenytoin, mephenytoin, phenytoin]	Decreased concentrations of cyclosporine.	CYP3A4 induction by Hydantoins
	HMG-CoA Reductase Inhibitors [fluvastatin, lovastatin,	Increased risk of rhabdomyolysis.	Inhibition of CYP3A4 mediated HMG-CoA Reductase Inhibitors

DRUG	DRUG INTERACTION	EFFECT	MECHANISM OF INTERACTION
	simvastatin]		metabolism by Cyclosporine
	Imipenem/ Cilastatin	Increased CNS adverse effects of both drugs (confusion, agitation, tremor).	undefined
	Macrolide Antibiotics [azithromycin, clarithromycin, erythromycin, troleandomycin]	Increased concentrations of cyclosporine.	Inhibition of CYP isoenzyme responsible for cyclosporine metabolism
	Metoclopramide	Increased concentrations of cyclosporine.	The prokinetic effect of metoclopramide on GI tract, which result in more rapid transport of cyclosporine
	Nefazodone	Increased concentrations of cyclosporine.	Inhibtion of CYP3A4 mediated cyclosporine metabolism by Nefazodone
	Nicardipine	Increased concentrations of Calcium channel blockers.	Inhibition of CYP3A4 by Cyclosporine decrease Calcium channel blockers metabolism
	NSAIDs	Enhance the	Inhibition of PG

DRUG	DRUG INTERACTION	EFFECT	MECHANISM OF INTERACTION
		nephrotoxic effect of cyclosporine, and increase serum concentration of cyclosporine	synthesis especially in kidney. The mechanism of increase in concentration is unclear
	Orlistat	decrease concentrations of cyclosporine.	Decrease in cyclosporine absorption from GIT (recommended separation of dose at bleast by 2 hours between tow drugs)
	Quinolones [ciprofloxacin, norfloxacin]	Increased risk of nephrotoxicity.	Inhibition of CYP3A4
	Rifamycins [rifabutin, rifampin]	Decreased concentrations of cyclosporine.	Induction of CYP3A4 by rifamycins
	Serotonin Reuptake Inhibitors	Increased concentrations of cyclosporine.	Inhibition of CYP3A4 mediated cyclosporine metabolism by SSRIs
	Sirolimus,	Increase serum concentration of sirolimus. Enhance adverse/ toxic effect of Cyclosporine, increase in risk of	cyclosporine inhibition of P-glycoprotein, which is responsible for the active efflux of sirolimus

DRUG	DRUG INTERACTION	EFFECT	MECHANISM OF INTERACTION
		calcineurin inhibitor—induce hemolytic uremic syndrume/ thrombotic thrombocytopenic purpura/ thrombotic microangiopathy	
	Sulfonamides [sulfadiazine, sulfamethoxazole , trimethoprim/ sulfamethoxazole]	Decreased effects of cyclosporine. Increased risk of nephrotoxicity with oral sulfonamides.	undefined
	Verapamil	Increased concentrations of Calcium channel blockers.	Inhibition of CYP3A4 by Cyclosporine decrease Calcium channel blockers metabolism

Mycophenolate mofetil

DRUG	DRUG INTERACTION	EFFECT	MECHANISM OF INTERACTION
Mycophenolate mofetil	Clindamycin	Decrease serum conc.of active metabolite of mycophenolate	Clindamycin kill glucuronidase— producing bacteria in GIT that mediate the metabolism of mycophenolate

DRUG	DRUG INTERACTION	EFFECT	MECHANISM OF INTERACTION
	metronidazol	Decrease serum concentration of mycophenolate (decrease effectiveness)	Inhibition of active metabolite formation of mycophenolate

Sirolimus

DRUG	DRUG INTERACTION	EFFECT	MECHANISM OF INTERACTION
Sirolimus	Azole Antifungals [fluconazole, itraconazole, ketoconazole, voriconazole]	Increased concentrations of sirolimus.	Inhibition of CYP3A4 mediated tacrolimus metabolism by Azole Antifungals
	Cyclosporine	Increase serum concentration of sirolimus. Enhance adverse/ toxic effect of Cyclosporine, increase in risk of calcineurin inhibitor—induce hemolytic uremic syndrume/ thrombotic thrombocytopenic purpura/ thrombotic microangiopathy	cyclosporine inhibition of P-glycoprotein, which is responsible for the active efflux of sirolimus
	Diltiazem	Increased	Inhibition of

DRUG	DRUG INTERACTION	EFFECT	MECHANISM OF INTERACTION
		concentrations of sirolimus.	CYP3A4 by diltiazem

Tacrolimus

DRUG	DRUG INTERACTION	EFFECT	MECHANISM OF INTERACTION
Tacrolimus	Azole Antifungals [fluconazole, itraconazole, ketoconazole, miconazole, voriconazole]	Increased concentrations of tacrolimus.	Inhibition of CYP3A4 mediated tacrolimus metabolism by Azole Antifungals
	azathioprine	Enhance the adverse/ toxic effect of Azathioprine (risk of infection, lymphoma, and skin malignancy	Augmentation of immunosupprssion
	Caspofungin	Decreased concentrations of tacrolimus.	undefined
	Diltiazem	Increased concentrations of tacrolimus.	Inhibition of CYP3A4 by diltiazem
	Hydantoins [fosphenytoin, phenytoin]	Decreased concentrations of tacrolimus.	Induction of CYP3A4 mediated tacrolimus metabolism by phenytoin.

DRUG	DRUG INTERACTION	EFFECT	MECHANISM OF INTERACTION
		Increased concentrations of phenytoin.	The mechanism of increase phenytoin concentration is unclear
	Macrolide antibiotics (clarithromycin, erythromycin, telithromycin)	Increased serum concentrations of tacrolimus.	inhibition of CYP3A4 by macrolides
	Nifedipine	Increased concentrations of tacrolimus.	Inhibition of CYP3A4 by Nifedipine
	Rifamycins [rifabutin, rifampin, rifapentine]	Decreased concentrations of tacrolimus.	CYP3A4 induction by rifamycins

MISCELLANEOUS AGENTS

Ergot Alkaloids[dihydroergotamine, ergotamine, methysergide}

DRUG	DRUG INTERACTION	EFFECT	MECHANISM OF INTERACTION
Ergot Alkaloids	Beta-Blockers [carteolol, nadolol, penbutolol, pindolol, propranolol, timolol]	Increased risk of ergot toxicity (peripheral ischemia, gangrene).	unknown, but may involve blockade of beta-2-mediated (i.e., sympathetic) vasodilatation. In addition, beta-1 blockade reduces

DRUG	DRUG INTERACTION	EFFECT	MECHANISM OF INTERACTION
			cardiac output, which can diminish blood flow and exacerbate ergot-induced vasospasm. Peripheral ischemia, hypertension with chest pain, gangrene resulting in surgical amputation, and migraine exacerbation have been described in suspected cases of the interaction.
	indinavir	Increased risk of ergot toxicity (peripheral ischemia, peripheral vasospasm).	CYP3A4 inhibition by indinavir
	Macrolide Antibiotics [clarithromycin, erythromycin, troleandomycin]	Acute ergotism (peripheral ischemia).	inhibition of CYP3A4 by Clarithromycin
	Nitrates [amyl nitrite, isosorbide dinitrate, nitroglycerin]	Increased standing systolic blood pressure. Pharmacologic antagonism between dihydroergotamine and nitroglycerin may decrease	Pharmacologic antagonism between dihydroergotamine and nitroglycerin

DRUG	DRUG INTERACTION	EFFECT	MECHANISM OF INTERACTION
		antianginal effects of nitroglycerin.	
	NNRT Inhibitors [delavirdine, efavirenz]	Increased risk of ergot toxicity (peripheral ischemia, peripheral vasospasm).	Inhibition of CYP3A4 mediated ergot metabolism by NNRT Inhibitors
	Protease Inhibitors [amprenavir, indinavir, nelfinavir, ritonavir, saquinavir]	Increased risk of ergot toxicity (peripheral ischemia, peripheral vasospasm).	Inhibition of CYP3A4 by Delavirdine that reduce ergot metabolism
	Sibutramine,	Increased risk of serotonin syndrome (CNS irritability, shivering, myoclonus, altered consciousness).	Sibutramine inhibit serotonin reuptake, augment serotonergic effect of Ergot Alkaloids
	Voriconazole	Increased risk of ergot toxicity (peripheral ischemia, peripheral vasospasm).	Inhibition of CYP3A4 mediated ergot metabolism by Voriconazole

Estrogens

[chlorotrianisene, conjugated estrogens, diethylstilbesterol, esterified estrogens, estradiol, estriol, estrogenic substance, estrone, estropipate,ethinyl estradiol,mestranol, quinestrol]

DRUG	DRUG INTERACTION	EFFECT	MECHANISM OF INTERACTION
Estrogens	Barbiturates [amobarbital, aprobarbital, butabarbital, butalbital, mephobarbital, pentobarbital, phenobarbital, primidone, secobarbital, thiamylal]	Decreased concentrations of estrogen (contraceptive failure).	Barbiturates induce metabolism of Estrogens
	Corticosteroids (Betamethason, Corticotropin, Cortisone, Cosyntropin, Dexamethasone Fludrocortisone, Hydrocortisone, Methylprednisolone, Prednisolone, Prednisone, Triamcinolone,),	Increased effects of Corticosteroids.	1.change in Corticosteroids metabolism 2.change in the ability of Corticosteroids to pined to proteins
	Hydantoins [ethotoin, fosphenytoin, mephenytoin, phenytoin]	Decreased concentrations of estrogen.	Hydantoins induce metabolism of Estrogens

DRUG	DRUG INTERACTION	EFFECT	MECHANISM OF INTERACTION
	Corticosteroids (Betamethason, Corticotropin, Cortisone, Cosyntropin, Dexamethason, Fludrocortisone, Hydrocortisone, Methylprednisolone, Prednisolone, Prednisone, Triamcinolone,)	Increased effects of Corticosteroids.	1.change in Corticosteroids metabolism 2.change in the ability of Corticosteroids to pined to proteins
	Penicillins	Diminish the therapeutic effect of oral contraceptive (estrogens)	Penicillins reduce gut bacteria which are important for hydrolysis of conjucated estrogen
	Protease Inhibitors [amprenavir, indinavir, nelfinavir, ritonavir, saquinavir]	Loss of contraceptive efficacyof ethinyl estradiol.	involve ritonavir induction of glucuronosyltransferase and/or CYP450 hydroxylation. Since estrogens and progestins may share common routes of metabolism
	Rifamycins [rifabutin, rifampin, rifapentine]	Decreased concentrations of estrogen	Induction of CYP3A4 by rifamycins

DRUG	DRUG INTERACTION	EFFECT	MECHANISM OF INTERACTION
	thyroxine	Decreased serum concentrations of free thyroxine.\n\nIncreased serum concentrations of thyrotropin.	Estrogens are known to increase serum thyroid-binding globulin concentration in a dose-dependent manner. Consequently, there may be a reduction in unbound, or free, thyroxine available for hormone activity, which, in turn, leads to an increase in serum thyrotropin concentration

Ethanol

DRUG	DRUG INTERACTION	EFFECT	MECHANISM OF INTERACTION
Ethanol	Acetaminophen,	Increased risk of acetaminophen-induced hepatotoxicity.	induction of hepatic microsomal enzymes during chronic alcohol use, which may result in accelerated metabolism of acetaminophen and increased production of potentially hepatotoxic metabolites

DRUG	DRUG INTERACTION	EFFECT	MECHANISM OF INTERACTION
	Alfentanil	additive CNS-depression and impairment of judgment, thinking, and psychomotor skills.	additive CNS-effects
	Barbiturates [amobarbital, butabarbital, butalbital, mephobarbital, pentobarbital, phenobarbital, primidone, secobarbital]	Additive CNS effects including impaired coordination, sedation, and death with acute ethanol ingestion (potentially fatal).	The mechanism is related to inhibition of microsomal enzymes acutely and induction of hepatic microsomal enzymes chronically
	Benzodiazepines [alprazolam, chlordiazepoxide, clorazepate, diazepam, estazolam, flurazepam, halazepam, lorazepam, midazolam, oxazepam, prazepam, quazepam,	Additive CNS depressione with acute ethanol ingestion.	Additive CNS effects with acute ethanol ingestion

DRUG	DRUG INTERACTION	EFFECT	MECHANISM OF INTERACTION
	temazepam, triazolam]		
	Cephalosporins [cefamandole, cefoperazone, ceforanide, cefonicid, cefotetan moxalactam]	Disulfuram-like reaction.	These agents contain an N-methylthiotetrazole (NMTT) side chain that may inhibit aldehyde dehydrogenase (ALDH) similar to disulfiram. Following ingestion of alcohol, inhibition of ALDH results in increased concentration of acetaldehyde, the accumulation of which produces an unpleasant physiologic response referred to as the 'disulfiram reaction.
	Chloral Hydrate	CNS depression.	Additive CNS depression
	Chlorpropamide	disulfiram-like reaction (flushing, headache, and nausea)	inhibits aldehyde dehydrogenase
	Disulfiram	Flushing, tachycardia, bronchospasm, sweating,	Disulfiram inhibits aldehyde dehydrogenase, the enzyme

DRUG	DRUG INTERACTION	EFFECT	MECHANISM OF INTERACTION
		nausea, and vomiting. May progress to death.	responsible for conversion of acetyldehyde in to carbon dioxide. Acetaldehyde accumulation result in toxic reaction
	Glutethimide	Additive CNS depression.	Additive CNS effects with acute ethanol ingestion
	Insulin,	Increased hypoglycemic effects of insulin.	Ethanol cause inhibition of gluconeogenesis as well as the counterregulatory response to hypoglycemia
	Meprobamate	Increased CNS depression.	Additive CNS effects with acute ethanol ingestion
	Metronidazole	Disulfiram-like reaction.	Inhibition of acetaldehyde dehydrogenase by metronidazol
	Phenothiazines [acetophenazin, chlorpromazine, fluphenazine,	Increased CNS depression and psychomotor impairment.	Additive CNS effects with acute ethanol ingestion

DRUG	DRUG INTERACTION	EFFECT	MECHANISM OF INTERACTION
	mesoridazine, perphenazine, prochlorperazine, promazine, promethazine, thioridazine, trifluoperazine, triflupromazine, trimeprazine]		
	Sulfonylureas [acetohexamide, chlorpropamide, glipizide, glyburide, tolazamide, tolbutamide]	Prolonged hypoglycemia. Disulfiram-like reaction when taken with chlorpropamide.	inhibition of gluconeogenesis and inhibition of the counterregulatory response to hypoglycemia.
	Verapamil	Increase therapeutic/toxic effect of verapamil	Inhibition of CYP3A4 by Ethanol

Levothyroxine

DRUG	DRUG INTERACTION	EFFECT	MECHANISM OF INTERACTION
Levothyroxine	Cholestyramine	Decreased GI	Cholestyramine bind

DRUG	DRUG INTERACTION	EFFECT	MECHANISM OF INTERACTION
		absorption of levothyroxine.	Levothyroxine in GIT that reduce its absorption
	digoxin	Increased concentrations of digoxin.	The clearance of digitalis glycosides may be reduced when a euthyroid state is achieved after the addition of antithyroid agents.
	Estrogens [conjugated estrogens, esterified estrogens, estradiol, estrone, estropipate, esthinyl estradiol, mestranol]	Decreased serum concentrations of free thyroxine. Increased serum concentrations of thyrotropin.	Estrogens are known to increase serum thyroid-binding globulin concentration in a dose-dependent manner. Consequently, there may be a reduction in unbound, or free, thyroxine available for hormone activity, which, in turn, leads to an increase in serum thyrotropin concentration
	Iron Salts (Oral) [ferrous fumarate, ferrous gluconate, ferrous sulfate, ironpolysaccharide]	Decreased GI absorption of levothyroxine.	Formation of poorly absorbed complex
	Sucralfate	Decreased GI absorption of levothyroxine.	Formation of poorly absorbed complex

DRUG	DRUG INTERACTION	EFFECT	MECHANISM OF INTERACTION
	Theophylline,	Decreased theophylline concentrations in hyperthyroid patients; returns to normal once euthyroid state achieved.	Increase in theophylline metabolism in hyperthyroid patients. Decrease theophylline metabolism in hypothyroid patient
	Warfarin,	Increased effects of warfarin.	Thyroid hormones increase the catabolism of the clotting factors dependent on vitamin K. The hypoprothrombinemic response to oral anticoagulants may be enhanced

Metyrapone

DRUG	DRUG INTERACTION	EFFECT	MECHANISM OF INTERACTION
Metyrapone	Cyproheptadine	Decreased pituitary-adrenal response to metyrapone.	may involve the antiserotonergic effect of cyproheptadine.
	Hydantoins [ethotoin, fosphenytoin, mephenytoin, phenytoin]	Decreased pituitary-adrenal response to metyrapone.	Induction of metyrapone metabolism

Quinine

DRUG	DRUG INTERACTION	EFFECT	MECHANISM OF INTERACTION
Quinine	clarthromycin	Increase risk of elevated quinine serum level and potential adverse cardiac effects and QTc-prolongation of quinine	The precise mechanism is unknown, but likely result from inhibition of quinine metabolisim by CYP3A4 inhibitors
	Digoxin	Increased concentrations/ toxic effect of digoxin.	Quinine reduce clearance (ninrenal) of digoxin
	fluconazole	Increase risk of ventricular fibrillation	Augmentation of QTc—prolongation by both drugs
	Rifamycins [rifabutin, rifampin, rifapentine]	Decreased concentrations of quinine.	Protein displacement of Quinine and increase clearance and metabolism Quinine
	Warfarin,	Enhance the anticoagulant effects of warfarin.	unknown

Sibutramine

DRUG	DRUG INTERACTION	EFFECT	MECHANISM OF INTERACTION
Sibutramine	Dextromethorphan	Increased risk of serotonin syndrome (CNS irritability, shivering, myoclonus, altered consciousness).	Dextromethorphan Increase serotonin activity, Sibutramine inhibit serotonin reuptake
	Ergot Alkaloids	Increased risk of serotonin syndrome (CNS irritability, shivering, myoclonus, altered consciousness).	Sibutramine inhibit serotonin reuptake, augment serotonergic effect of Ergot Alkaloids
	Lithium	Increased risk of serotonin syndrome (CNS irritability, shivering, myoclonus, altered consciousness).	Sibutramine inhibit serotonin reuptake and litium have serotonin agonist
	MAO Inhibitors [isocarboxazid, phenelzine, tranylcypromine]	Increased risk of serotonin syndrome (CNS irritability, shivering, myoclonus, altered consciousness).	Sibutramine inhibit serotonin reuptake. MAOI reduce serotonin metabolism
	Meperidine	Increased risk of serotonin syndrome (CNS	Meperidine Increase serotonin activity,

DRUG	DRUG INTERACTION	EFFECT	MECHANISM OF INTERACTION
		irritability, shivering, myoclonus, altered consciousness).	Sibutramine inhibit serotonin reuptake
	Selective 5HT-1 Receptor Antagonists [almotriptan, naratriptan, rizatriptan, sumatriptan, zolmitriptan]	Increased risk of serotonin syndrome (CNS irritability, shivering, myoclonus, altered consciousness).	Selective 5HT-1 Receptor Antagonists Increase serotonin activity, Sibutramine inhibit serotonin reuptake
	Serotonin Reuptake Inhibitors [fluoxetine, fluvoxamine, nefazodone, paroxetine, sertraline, venlafaxine]	Increased risk of serotonin syndrome (CNS irritability, shivering, myoclonus, altered consciousness).	Additive effect on serotonin, Sibutramine inhibit serotonin reuptake that increase effect of Serotonin Reuptake Inhibitors
	Tryptophan	Increased risk of serotonin syndrome (CNS irritability, shivering, myoclonus, altered consciousness).	Tryptophan Increase serotonin activity, Sibutramine inhibit serotonin reuptake

INDEX

Alpha 1-Blockers (Prazosin, Doxazocin, Phenoxybenzamine, Phyntolamine, Tamsulosin, Terazosin)	78-79,82,97
Alprazolam	26,30,56,66,92,148,198-200,261
Alteplase	109,123-124
Aluminum Carbonate	43,235-236
Aluminum Hydroxide	21,43,235-236
Aluminum -Magnesium Hydroxide	21, 235-236
Aluminum Phosphate	43,235-236
Aluminum Salts [Aluminum Carbonate, Aluminum Hydroxide, Aluminum Phosphate, Attapulgite, Kaolin, Magaldrate]	43,235-236
Ambenonium	242
Amikacin	16-18,19,21,43,44,110,116,144
Amiloride	105
Aminoglutethimide	126
Aminoglycoside	16-18,21,43,44,110,116,144
Aminophylline	147-152
Aminoquinolines (Antimalarial) (Chloroquine, Hydroxychloroquine, Primaquine	110
Aminosalisylate	75
Amiodarone	37,56,61,62,98-100,103,105,110, 126,148,164,205,206,212,224, 228,247,
Amitriptyline	11,38,55,76,159,175,182,185, 189-191,234
Amlodipine	23,27,31,51,69,71,72,90-98,111, 115,165,171,232,236,237,248,250, 252

Antiarrhythmic Agents [Amiodarone, Bretylium, Disopyramide, Procainamide, Quinidine, Sotalol]	98-108
Anticholinesterases [Ambenonium, Edrophonium, Neostigmine, Pyridostigmine]	242
Anticoagulants [Anisidione, Dicumarol, Warfarin]	14,20,22,30,33,35,36,43,47,55,68, 75, 100, 108,119,120,126-135, 142, 145, 152,160,164, 165, 197,208, 211, 222, 225,226, 223,231, 234,246,266,267
ANTICONVULSANT	154-180
ANTIDEPRESSANTS	11,38,55,76,159,175,180-193,234
Antiemetics(5HT3 Antagonists) Alosetron, Ondansetron	50
Antifungal Agents (Azole Derivatives, Systemic)	25,30,66-74,107
ANTIHYPERTENSIVE DRUGS	76-97
Antimalarial	110
Antineoplastic Agents (Vinca Alkaloids)	26,110
Antineoplastic Agents [Bleomycin, Carmustine, Cyclophosphamide, Cytarabine, Doxorubicin, Methotrexate, Vincristine]	110
ANTIPARKINSON AGENT	153-154
ANTIPSYCHOTIC Agents	201-202
ANTIVIRAL AGENTS	56-65
Aprepitant	223
Aprobarbital	45,74,75,82,90,105,127,148, 194-197
ARTHRITIS AND GOUT AGENTS	141-147

Aspirin	12,15,75,123,125,133,135,140,146, 174,208-211,216,220,238,242
Atazanavir	55
Atenolol	21,51,76,78,82-84,87,102,105
Atovaquone	38
Atracurium	49,97
Attapulgite	43
Azathioprine	79,138,142,254
Azithromycin	23-25,130,229,250
Azole Antifungals [Fluconazole, Itraconazole, Ketoconazole Voriconazole Miconazole]	56,66-74,90,101,127,136,168,198, 2 00,202,204,219,223,228,224,245, 247,253,254,267
Bacampicillin	18,19-21,40,131,139,259
Barbiturates [Amobarbital, Aprobarbital, Butabarbital, Butalbital, Mephobarbital, Pentobarbital, Phenobarbital, Primidone, Secobarbital]	41,42,45,50,74,82,90,105,127,148, 173,194-198,213,242,258,261
BCG	16,19,38
Benazepril	79-81,144,167,191
Bendroflumethiazide	118,
Benzodiazepines, Oxidative Metabolism-Class [Alprazolam, Chlordiazepoxid, Clonazepam, Clorazepate, Diazepam, Estazolam, Flurazepam, Halazepam, Midazolam, Quazepam, Triazolam]	26,30,56,66,92,148,198-200,261
Benzphetamine	184-185
Benzthiazide	118,179,193,217,220
Bepridil	111

Beta-Blockers [Acebutolol, Atenolol, Betaxolol, Bisoprolol, Carteolol, Esmolol, Metoprolol, Nadolol, Penbutolol, Pindolol, Propranolol, Sotalol, Timolol]	76,78,82-90,95,102,115,116,144, 148,161,194,215,232,255
Betamethasone	23,27,34,52,161,166,194,209, 242-245,258,259
Betaxolol	76,78,82-84
Bile Acid Sequestrant (Cholestyramine, Colesevelam, Colestipol	39,98,111,117,128,173,207,225, 224-225,228,244,264
Bismuth Salts	38,123
Bismuth Subsalicylate	12,15,75,123,125,133,135,140,146, 174,208-211,216,220,238,242
Bisoprolol	15,78,82-84
Bleomycin	110
Bretylium	206
Bromocriptine	26,31
BRONCHODILATORS	147-152
Bumetanide	17,112,116-117
Bupropion	63,154,175-176,180
Buproprion	63,160
Buspirone	26,31,51,66,200-201
Busulfan	45
Butabarbital	45,74,75,82,90,105,127,148, 194-198,213,242,258,261
Butalbital	45,74,75,82,90,105,127,148, 194-198,213,242,258,261
Caffeine	36

Calcium Acetate	33,38,95,235-236,237
Calcium Carbonate	33,38,95, 235-236,240
Calcium Channel Blockers (Amlodipine, Diltiazem,Isradipine, Felodipine, Nicardipine, Nifedipine,Verapamil)	23,27,31,51,69,71,72,90-98,111, 165,171,232,236,237,248,250, 252
Calcium Chloride	95,235-236
Calcium Citrate	95,235-236
Calcium Glubionate	95,235-236
Calcium Gluconate	95,235-236
Calcium Glycerophosphate	95,235-236
Calcium Iodide	95,235-236
Calcium Lactate	95,235-236
Calcium Levulinate	95,235-236
Calcium Salts [Calcium Acetate, Calcium Carbonate, Calcium Chloride, Calcium Citrate, Calcium Glubionate, Calcium Gluconate, Calcium Glycerophosphate, Calcium Lactate, Calcium Levulinate, Tricalcium Phosphate]	95,235-236
Candesartan	81,177,191
Capreomycin	16
Captopril	79-81,144,176,191
Carbamazepine	14,26,31,41,49,91,96,127,149, 154-160.165,173,175,177,180, 183,185,189,191,194,202,215, 323,248
Carbenicillin	18,19-21,40,131,139,259
Carbonic Anhydrase Inhibitors [Acetazolamide, Dichlorphenamid, Methazolamide]	208

Cardio-Selective (Acebutolol, Atenolol, Betaxolol, Bisoprolol, Esmolol, Metoprolol, Nadolol)	82-84
CARDIOVASCULAR AGENTS	76-118
Carmustine	110
Carteolol	76,78,84-90,115,216,255
Carvedilol	76,78,84-90,115,216,255
Caspofungin	254
Cefamandole	16,21-23,127,262
Cefazolin	16, 21-23,127,262
Cefonicid	21-23,127,262
Cefoperazone	16, 21-23,127,262
Cefotaxime	16, 21-23
Cefotetan	16, 21-23,127,262
Cefoxitin	16, 21-23,127
Ceftazidime	16, 21-23
Ceftizoxime	16, 21-23
Ceftriaxone	16, 21-23,127
Cefuroxime	16, 21-23
Cephalosporins	16, 21-23,127,235,262
Cephalothin	16, 21-23
Cephapirin	16, 21-23
Cephradine	16, 21-23
Chloral Hydrate	262
Chloramphenicol	42-43,51,120,121,128,166,195, 219
Chlordiazepoxide	26,30,56,66,92,148,198-200,261

Chloroquine	110
Chlorothiazide	114,118,179,193,218,220
Chlorotrianisene	56,195,258-260
Chlorpromazine	88,89,203-204,205,213,263
Chlorpropamide	35,43,48,54,68,81,118,133,182,210, 218-224,264
Chlorthalidone	114,118,179,193,218,220
Cholestyramine	39,98,111,117,128,173,207, 224-225,228,244,264
Choline Salicylate	12,15,75,123,125,133,135,140,146, 174,208-211,216,220,238,242
Cilastatin	250
Cimetidine	14,57,82,91,94,102,103,128,149, 154,166,183,189,217,232-234,
Ciprofloxacin	25,33-38,60,90,100,101,104,107, 123,132,150,221,241,251
Cisapride	26,69,70,72
Cisplatin	17,116
Citolapram	145,159,183-187,189,204,234,269
Clarithromycin	23-30,34,51,65,112,130,135,142, 145,150,154,157,198,199,200, 211,230,243,250,255,256
Clindamycin	17,43-44,252
Clofibrate	129,226
Clomipramine	11,38,55,76,159,175,182,185, 189-191,234
Clonazepam	26,30,56,66,92,148,,198-200,261
Clonidine	76-77,83,189

Clopidogrel	27,49,51,58,69,70,72,125,136-137,183,239
Clorazepate	26,30,56,66,92,148,,198-200,261
Cloxacillin	18,19-21,40,131,139,259
Clozapine	63,183,201,202
Codeine	106,212
Colchicine	27,31,39,45,124,142-143,284
Colesevelam	39,98,111,117,128,173,207,225, 224-225,228,244,264
Colestipol	39,98,111,117,128,173,207,225, 224-225,228,244,264
Colistimethate	17
Conjugated Estrogens	20,51,52,56,57,63.162,168,195,196, 242,243, 258-260,265
Contraceptives (Progestins, Estrogens)	7,51,149,160,
Corticorelin	124
Corticosteroids [Betamethasone, Cortisone, Corticotropin, Desoxycorticosterone, Dexamethasone, Fludrocortisone, Hydrocortisone, Methylprednisolone, Paramethasone, Prednisolone, Prednisone, Triamcinolone]	23,27,34,52,161,166,194,209, 242-245,258,259
Corticotropin	23,27,34,52,161,166,194,209, 242-245,258,259
Cortisone	23,27,34,52,161,166,194,209, 242-245,258,259
Cosyntropin	23,27,34,52,161,166,194,209, 242-245,258,259

Cyanocobalamin	42,239
Cyclophosphamide	110
Cyclosporine	23,36,47,52,66,79,87,91,92,94,96, 98,111,119,142,145,155,167,183, 228,229,231,239,247-252,253
Cyproheptadine	183,266
Cytarabine	110
Danazol	155,247
Dapsone	44,47
Delavirdine	52,56,58-59,135,257
Demeclocycline	11,20,38-42,113,114,123,143,212, 225,236,241
Desflurane	87
Desipramine	11,38,55,76,159,175,182,185, 189-191,234
Desmopressin	177
Desoxycorticosterone	23,27,34,52,161,166,194,209, 242-245,258,259
Dexamethasone	23,27,34,52,161,166,194,209, 242-245,258,259
Dexfenfluramine	184-185
Dextroamphetamine	184-185
Dextromethorphan	268
Dextrothyroxine	128
Diazepam	26,30,56,66,92,148,,198-200,261
Diazoxide	167,219
Dichlorphenamid	208

Diclofenac	13,18,80,85,131,139,144-147,148, 192,250
Dicloxacillin	18,19-21,40,131,139,259
Dicumarol	14,20,22,30,33,35,36,43,47,55,68, 75, 100, 108,119,120,126-135, 142, 145, 152,160,164, 165, 197,208, 211, 222, 225,226, 223,231, 234,246,266,267
Didanosine	59-60,61,71,72,141
Diethylpropion	185
Diethylstilbesterol	20,51,52,56,57,63.162,168,195,196, 242,243, 258-260,265
Digoxin	7,11,12,15,17,24,39,69,71,73,96,98 , 104,106,110-115,117,118,138,146, 224,240,241,249,265,257
Dihydroergotamine	28,32,56,58,62,74,85,108,255-257, 268
Diltiazem	23,27,31,51,69,71,72,90-98,111, 115,16 5,171,232,236,237,248,250, 252
Dimercaprol	120,121
Dipyridamole	124,143
Discontinueephedrine	77
Disopyramide	28,32,37,52,55,101,167,206
Disulfiram	45,128,149,167,188,219,222,262, 263
Diuretics	116-118
Divalproex Sodium	55,159,161,163,164,172,173-175, 190,210,225
Dobutamine	77,190
Dopamine	77,190
Doxacurium	97
Doxazocin	78-79,82,97

Doxepin	38,55,76,115,159,175,182,185,187, 189-191,243
Doxorubicin	110
Doxycycline	11,20,38-42,113,114,123,143,212, 225,236,241
Dronedarone	184
Dyphylline	147-153
Edrophonium	242
Efavirenz	257
Enalapril	47,79-81,120,144,138,141,215, 218,247
Enflurane	87
Enoxaparin	136
Epinephrine	77,84,85,115-116,181,190,216
Eplerenone	28,39,45
Eprosartan	81,177,191
Ergot Alkaloids [Dihydroergotamine, Ergotamine, Methysergide	28,32,56,58,62,74,85,108,255-257, 268
Ergotamine	28,32,56,58,62,74,85,108,255-257, 268
Erythromycin	14,23-33,34,52,112,130,143,150, 155,157,199,201,211,230,243,250, 255,256
Escitalopram	145,159,183-187,189,204,234,269
Esmolol	76,82-90,102,115,116,144,148, 161,194,215,232,255
Esomeprazole	67,122,136,137,138,210,230, 237-239
Estazolam	26,30,56,66,92,148,198-200,261
Esterified Estrogens	20,51,52,56,57,63.162,168,195,196, 242,243, 258-260,265

Esthinyl Estradiol	20,51,52,56,57,63.162,168,195,196, 242,243, 258-260,265
Estrogens [Chlorotrianisene, Conjugated Estrogens, Diethylstilbesterol, Esterified Estrogens, Estradiol, Estrone, Estropipate, Ethinyl Estradiol, Quinestrol]	20,51,52,56,57,63.162,168,195,196, 242,243, 258-260,265
Estrone	20,51,52,56,57,63.162,168,195,196, 242,243, 258-260,265
Estropipate	20,51,52,56,57,63.162,168,195,196, 242,243, 258-260,265
Ethacrynic Acid	17,112,16-17,225,227
Ethanol	22,45,96,162,196,199,203,207,211, 216,219,222,260-264
Ethinyl Estradiol	20,51,52,56,57,63.162,168,195,196, 242,243, 258-260,265
Ethotoin	7,12,14,36,37,41,42,43,46,48,50 , 53,54,70,71,73,92,94,99,101,103 , 106,125,128,132,150,153,158, 164-173,174,186,188,197,198,207,214, 233, 241,243,245,249,254,255,258, 266
Ethotoinfosphenytoin	7,12,14,36,37,41,42,43,46,48,50 , 53,54,70,71,73,92,94,99,101,103 , 106,125,128,132,150,153,158, 164-173,174,186,188,197,198,207,214, 233, 241,243,245,249,254,255,258, 266
Etodolac	13,18,80,85,131,139,144-147,148, 192,250
Etoposide	249
Everolimus	45
Famotidine	73,231-232
Felbamate	168,174

Felodipine	23,27,31,51,69,71,72,90-98,111, 115,165,171,232,236,237,248,250, 252
Fenfluramine	184-185
Fenofibrate	129,226
Fenoprofen	13,18,80,85,131,139,144-147,148, 192,250
Fentanyl	39,98,212
Ferric Gluconate	120-123
Ferrous Fumarate	33,77, 120-123,153,235,238,265
Ferrous Gluconate	33,77, 120-123,153,235,238,265
Ferrous Sulfate	33,77, 120-123,153,235,238,265
Ferrousfumarate	33,77, 120-123,153,235,238,265
Fibric Acids [Clofibrate, Fenofibrate, Gemfibrozil]	129,226
Flecainide	57,64,101
Flubiprofen	13,18,80,85,131,139,144-147,148, 192,250
Fluconazole	56,66-74,90,101,127,136,168,198, 200,202,204,219,223,228,224,245, 247,253,254,267
Fludrocortisone	23,27,34,52,161,166,194,209, 242-245,258,259
Fluoxetine	145,159,178,182,183-192,213,234, 251,257,268,269
Fluoxymesterone	126
Fluphenazine	37,88,89,188,203-206,213,263
Flurazepam	26,30,56,66,92,148,,198-200,261
Fluvastatin	24,53,67,93,96,98,99,130,224,226, 227,228-231,238,249

Glyburide	35,43,48,54,68,81,118,133,182,210, 218-224,264
Griseofulvin	74-75,129,162,196
Halazepam	26,30,56,66,92,148,,198-200,261
Haloperidol	52,67,156,177,192,202
Halothane	87,149
Heparin	109,124-125,209
Histamine H2-Antagonists[Cimetidine, Famotidine, Nizatidine, Ranitidine]	73,231-234
HMG-Coa Reductase Inhibitors [Fluvastatin, Lovastatin, Simvastatin Pravastatin, Rosuvastatin, Atorvastatin]	24,53,67,93,96,98,99,130,224,226, 227,228-231,238,249
Hydantoins [Ethotoin, Fosphenytoin, Mephenytoin, Phenytoin]	7,12,14,36,37,41,42,43,46,48,50 , 53,54,70,71,73,92,94,99,101,103 , 106,125,128,132,150,153,158, 164-173,174,186,188,197,198,207,214, 233, 241,243,245,249,254,255,258, 266
Hydralazine	83,161
Hydrochlorothiazide	114,118,179,193,217,220
Hydrocortisone	23,27,34,52,161,166,194,209, 242-245,258,259
Hydroflumethiazide	114,118,179,193,217,220
Hydrogen Iodide	178,192
Hydroxychloroquine	110
HYPOGLYCEMIC AGENTS	215-224
HYPOLIPIDEMIC AGENTS	224-231
Ibuprofen	13,18,80,85,131,139,144-147,148, 192,250
Imipenem	250

Indapamide	114,118,179,193,217,220
Indinavir	53,56-57,60,61-62,67,101,108,200, 201,256,257,259
Indomethacin	13,18,80,85,131,139,144-147,148, 192,250
Inhalation Anesthetics [Desflurane, Enflurane, Halothane, Isoflurane, Sevoflurane]	87
Insulin	34, 80,85,181,209,215-216,263
Iodide Salts [Calcium Iodide, Hydrogen Iodide, Iodide, Iodinated Glycerol, Iodine, Potassium Iodide, Sodium Iodide]	178,192
Iodinated Contrast Materials, IV	217
Iodinated Glycerol	178,192
Irbesartan	81,177,191
Iron Dextran	80,120-121
Iron Polysaccharide	33,77,121-123,153,235
Iron Products	42,120-123
Iron Salts (IV) [Iron Dextran, Ferric Gluconate, Iron Sucrose]	120-121
Iron Salts (Oral) [Ferrous Fumarate, Ferrous Sulfate, Iron Polysaccharide]	121-123
Iron Sucrose	120-121
Iron-Dextran Complex	80, 120-121
Isocarboxazid	77,115,153,157,175,180-182,184, 190,212,216,219,268
Isoflurane	87
Isoniazid	49-50,55,136,156,169

Isosorbide Dinitrate	108-109,256
Isradipine	23,27,31,51,69,71,72,90-98,111, 115,16 5,171,232,236,237,248,250, 252
Itraconazole	56,60,66-72,90,107,111,127,169,198, 200,202,204,219,228,244, 247,253,254
Kanamycin	16-18,19,21,43,44,110,116,144
Kaolin	43
Kayexalate	236,240
Ketoconazole	56,60,63,66-74,90,127,169,198, 2 00,202,219,228,231,232,235,238, 244,245,247,253,254
Ketoprofen	13,18,80,85,131,139,144-147,148, 192,250
Ketorolac	13,18,80,85,131,139,144-147,148, 192,250
Labetalol	48-87,
Lamotrigine	157,160-161,174
Lansoprazole	67,122,136,137,138,210,230,237-239
Leukotriene Inhibitors	152
Levamisole	130
Levodopa	9,121,153-154,170,176,181,240
Levofloxacin	25,33-38,60,90,100,101,104,107, 123,132,150,221,241,251
Levothyroxine	114,122,134,151,225,241,264-266
Lidocaine	87,88,89,102,206,232
Liothyronine	114,122,134,151,225,241,264-266
Liotrix	114,122,134,151,225,241,264-266
Lisinopril	47,79-81,120,144,138,141,215, 218,247

Lithium	7,77,80,81,118,145,157,176-193, 202,268
Loop Diuretics-Class [Bumetanide, Ethacrynic Acid, Furosemide, Torsemide	17,112,16-17,225,227
Loratadine	99
Lorazepam	26,30,56,66,92,148,,198-200,261
Losartan	81,177,191
Lovastatin	24,67,99,130,228-231,238,249
Macrolide Antibiotics(Clarithromycine, Erythomycine, Telithromycine) Azithromycin, Spiromycim	23-33,91,112,130,150,157,199,200, 229,243,250,255,256
Magaldrate	43
Magnesium Hydroxide	21,33,38,73,107,122,235-237.240
Magnesium Salicylate	12,15,75,123,125,133,135,140,146, 174,208-211,216,220,238,242
MAO Inhibitors[Isocarboxazid, Phenelzine, Selegiline, Tranylcypromine]	77,115,153,157,175,180-182,184, 190,212,216,219,268
Mazindol	184-185
Mebendazole	46
Meclofenamate	13,18,80,85,131,139,144-147,148, 192,250
Mefenamic Acid	13,18,80,85,131,139,144-147,148, 192,250
Meloxicam	13,18,80,85,131,139,144-147,148, 192,250
Meperidine	64,181,205,212-213,268
Mephentermine	77,190

Mephenytoin	7,12,14,36,37,41,42,43,46,48,50 ,53,54,70,71,73,92,94,99,101,103 ,106,125,128,132,150,153,158, 164-173,174,186,188,197,198,207,214, 233, 241,243,245,249,254,255,258, 266
Mephobarbital	45,74,75,82,90,105,127,148, 194-198,213,242,258,261
Meprobamate	263
Mesoridazine	37,88,89,188,203-206,213,263
Mestranol	20,51,52,56,57,63.162,168,195,196, 242,243, 258-260,265
Metaraminol	77-78,190
Metformin	22,118,217-218,233
Methacycline	11,20,38-42,113,114,123,143,212, 225,236,241
Methadone	53,162,170,186,196,213-214
Methamphetamin	184-185
Methazolamide	208
Methenamine	48
Methicillin	18,19-21,40,131,139,259
Methimazole	88,89,114,134,151
Methotrexate	12,15,19,36,39,48,110,138-140, 145,150,178,210
Methotrimeprazine	37,88,89,188,203-206,213,263
Methoxamine	78,190
Methyclothiazide	114,118,179,193,217,220
Methyldopa	77-78,122,178,181
Methylphenidate	153

Methylprednisolone	23,27,34,52,161,166,194,209, 242-245,258,259
Methyltestosterone	119-120
Methyltestosterone/ Testosterone	119-120
Methysergide	28,32,56,58,62,74,85,108,255-257, 268
Metoclopramide	112,153,239-240,250
Metolazone	114,118,179,193,217,220
Metoprolol	51,76,78,82-90,102,104,105,115, 116,161
Metronidazole	44-47,130,136,170,196,263
Metyrapone	170,266
Mexiletine	103,150,170
Mezlocillin	18,19-21,40,131,139,259
Miconazole	56,66-74,90,101,127,136,168,198, 200,202,204,219,223,228,224,245, 247,253,254,267
Midazolam	26,30,56,66,92,148,,198-200,261
Minocycline	11,20,38-42,113,114,123,143,212, 225,236,241
Mivacurium	97
Moexipril	47,79-81,120,144,138,141,215, 218,247
Monoamine Oxidase Inhibitors(MAO Inhibitors): Isocarboxazid, Phenelzine, Selegiline, Tranylcypromine	77,115,153,157,175,180-182,184, 190,212,216,219,268
Moricizine	233
Morphine	13,53214
Moxifloxacin	25,33-38,60,90,100,101,104,107, 123,132,150,221,241,251

Mycophenolate Mofetil	252-253
Nabumetone	13,18,80,85,131,139,144-147,148, 192,250
Nadolol	76,78,82-90,95,102,115,116, 216, 255
Nafcillin	18,19-21,40,131,139,259
Nalidixic Acid	25,33-38,60,90,100,101,104,107, 123,132,150,221,241,251
Nandrolone Decanoate	119,127
Naproxen	13,18,80,85,131,139,144-147,148, 192,250
Narcotic	211-215
Nefazodone	145,159,178,182,183-192,213,234, 251,257,268,269
Nelfinavir	53,56- 67,101,108,200, 201,256,257,259
Neomycin	16-18,19,21,43,44,110,116,144
Neostigmine	242
Nicardipine	23,27,31,51,69,71,72,90-98,111, 115,16 5,171,232,236,237,248,250, 252
Nifedipine	23,27,31,51,69,71,72,90-98,111, 115,16 5,171,232,236,237,248,250, 252
Nislodipine	23,27,31,51,69,71,72,90-98,111, 115,16 5,171,232,236,237,248,250, 252
Nisoldipine	23,27,31,51,69,71,72,90-98,111, 115,16 5,171,232,236,237,248,250, 252
Nitrates [Amyl Nitrite, Isosorbide Dinitrate, Isosorbide Mononitrate Nitroglycerin]	108-109,256
Nitredipine	23,27,31,51,69,71,72,90-98,111, 115,16 5,171,232,236,237,248,250, 252
Nitroglycerin	108-109,256

Oxtriphylline	93,147-152
Oxymetholone	127
Oxytetracycline	11,20,38-42,113,114,123,143,212, 225,236,241
PAIN MEDICATIONS	207-215
Pancuronium	49,97
Pantoprazole	67,122,136,137,138,210,230, 237-239
Paramethasone	23,27,34,52,161,166,194,209, 242-245,258,259
Paroxetine	145,159,178,182,183-192,213,234, 251,257,268,269
Penbutolol	76,78,82-90,95,102,115, 148, 216,232,255
Penicillamine	113,122
Penicillin G	18,19-21,40,131,139,259
Penicillin G	18,19-21,40,131,139,259
Penicillin V	18,19-21,40,131,139,259
Penicillins	18,19-21,40,131,139,259
Pentobarbital	45,74,75,82,90,105,127,148, 194-198,213,242,258,261
Perindopril	47,79-81,120,144,138,141,215, 218,247
Perphenazine	37,88,89,188,203-206,213,263
Phendimetrazine	184-185
Phenelzine	77,115,153,157,175,180-182,184, 190,212,216,219,268
Phenmetrazine	184-185
Phenobarbital	45,74,75,82,90,105,127,148, 194-198,213,242,258,261

Polythiazide	114,118,179,193,217,220
Potassium Citrate	40,179,193,222
Potassium Iodide	178,192
Potassium-Sparing Diuretics	14, 81,113
Praziquantel	233
Prazosin	78-79,82,97
Prednisolone	23,27,34,52,161,166,194,209, 242-245,258,259
Prednisone	23,27,34,52,161,166,194,209, 242-245,258,259
Primaquine	110
Primidone	45,74,75,82,90,105,127,148,194-198,213,242,258,261
Probenecid	12,15,22,44,65,139,146,210
Probucol	228,248
Procainamide	37,48,99,103-104,206,234
Prochlorperazine	37,88,89,188,203-206,213,263
Progestins	51,160
Promazine	37,88,89,188,203-206,213,263
Promethazine	37,88,89,188,203-206,213,263
Propafenone	83,104-105,107,113
Propoxyphene	64,158,215
Propranolol	76,78,82-90,95,102,115,116,144, 148,161,194,215,232,255
Propylthiouracil	88,89,114,134,151

Protease Inhibitors [Amprenavir, Indinavir, Nelfinavir, Ritonavir, Saquinavir]	53,56- 67,101,108,200, 201,256,257,259
Proton Pump Inhibitors [Esomeprazole, Lansoprazole, Omeprazole, Pantoprazole, Rabeprazole]	67,122,136,137,138,210,230, 237-239
Protriptyline	38,55,76,115,159,175,182,185,187, 189-191,243
Pyridostigmine	242
Pyridoxine	154
Quazepam	26,30,56,66,92,148,,198-200,261
Quinapril	47,79-81,120,144,138,141,215, 218,247
Quinethazone	114,118,179,193,217,220
Quinidine	12,15,37,54,57,62,68,83,93,97,99 , 104,105-108,113,132,163,171,197, 206,212,234,235,241
Quinine Derivatives [Quinidine, Quinine]	12,15,37,54,57,62,68,83,93,97,99 , 104,105-108,113,132,163,171,197, 206,212,234,235,241
Quinolones	12,15,37,54,57,62,68,83,93,97,99 , 104,105-108,113,132,163,171,197, 206,212,234,235,241
Rabeprazole	67,122,136,137,137,210,230, 237-239
Ranitidine	73,231-232
Retinoic Acid Derivative	40
Rifabutin	42,50-55,62,67,92,107,132,151, 1 71,190,201,202,214,220,230,243, 251,255,259,267
Rifampin	42,50-55,62,67,92,107,132,151, 1 71,190,201,202,214,220,230,243, 251,255,259,267

Rifamycins [Rifabutin, Rifampin, Rifapentine]	42,50-55,62,67,92,107,132,151, 1 71,190,201,202,214,220,230,243, 251,255,259,267
Rifapentine	42,50-55,62,67,92,107,132,151, 1 71,190,201,202,214,220,230,243, 251,255,259,267
Ritonavir	53,56- 67,101,108,200, 201,256,257,259
Rizatriptan	269
R-Warfarin	14,20,22,30,33,35,36,43,47,55,68, 75, 100, 108,119,120,126-135, 142, 145, 152,160,164, 165, 197,208, 211, 222, 225,226, 223,231, 234,246,266,267
Salicylates [Aspirin, Bismuth Subsalicylate, Choline Salicylate, Magnesium Salicylate, Salsalate, Sodium Salicylate, Sodium Thiosalicylate]	12,15,75,123,125,133,135,140,146, 174,208-211,216,220,238,242
Salmeterol	29,46,58,62,64
Saquinavir	53,56- 67,101,108,200, 201,256,257,259
Secobarbital	45,74,75,82,90,105,127,148,194-198,213,242,258,261
Sedatives [Barbiturates, Amobarbital, Butabarbital, Butalbital, Mephobarbital, Pentobarbital, Phenobarbital, Primidone, Secobarbital	45,74,75,82,90,105,127,148,194-198,213,242,258,261
SEDATIVES- HYPNOTICS AGENTS	180-182
Selective 5HT-1 Receptor Antagonists [Almotriptan, Naratriptan, Rizatriptan, Sumatriptan, Zolmitriptan]	269
Selegiline	77,115,153,157,175,180-182,184, 190,212,216,219,268
Inhibitors [Fluoxetine, Fluvoxamine, Paroxetine, Sertraline]	145,159,178,182,183-192,213,234, 251,257,268,269

Sertraline	145,159,171,178,182,183-192,188, 213,234, 251,257,268,269
Sevelamer	237
Sevoflurane	87
Sibutramine	178,182,184,192,213,257,268-269
Sildenafil	29,78,109
Simvastatin	24,53,67,93,96,98,99,130,224,226, 227,228-231,238,249
Sirolimus	68,93,251,253-254
Sodium Acetate	40,179,193,222
Sodium Bicarbonate	40,179,193,222
Sodium Citrate	40,179,193,222
Sodium Iodide	178,192
Sodium Polystyrene Sulfonate (Kayexalate)	236,240
Sodium Salicylate	12,15,75,123,125,133,135,140,146, 174,208-211,216,220,238,242
Sodium Thiosalicylate	12,15,75,123,125,133,135,140,146, 174,208-211,216,220,238,242
Sotalol	76,78,82-90,95,102,115,116,144, 148,161,194,215,232,255
Sparfloxacin	25,33-38,60,90,100,101,104,107, 123,132,150,221,241,251
Spironolactone	14,113
Stanozolol	126,127,247
Streptomycin	16-18,19,21,43,44,110,116,144
Sucralfate	34,40,108,113,133,171,241,256
Sulfadiazine	47,48,133,140,172,220,252

Sulfamethizole	47,48,133,140,172,220,252
Sulfamethoxazole	47,48,133,140,172,220,252
Sulfasalazine	47,48,133,140,172,220,252
Sulfinpyrazone	47,48,133,140,172,220,252
Sulfisoxazole	47,48,133,140,172,220,252
Sulfonamides [Sulfadiazine, Sulfamethizole, Sulfamethoxazole, Sulfasalazine, Sulfisoxazole, Trimethoprim/ Sulfamethoxazole]	47,48,133,140,172,220,252
Sulfonylureas [Acetohexamide, Chlorpropamide, Glimepride, Glipizide, Glyburide, Tolazamide, Tolbutamide]	35,43,48,54,68,81,118,133,182,210, 218-224,264
Sulindac	13,18,80,85,131,139,144-147,148, 192,250
Sumatriptan	269
Sympathomimetics [Amphetamine, Benzphetamine, Dextroamphetamine, Dexfenfluramine, Diethylpropion, Fenfluramine, Mazindol, Methamphetamin, Phendimetrazine, Phenmetrazine, Phentermine Pseudoephedrine,]	184-185
Tacrine	186
Tacrolimus	24,54,68,93,94,138,172,253,254-255
Tacrolimus(Topical)	138
Tamoxifen	54,58,102,134,176
Tamsulosin	78-79,82,97
Tapentadol	147
Tasalafil	29,78,109

Timolol	76,78,82-90,95,102,115,116,144, 148,161,194,215,232,255
Tobramycin	16-18,19,21,43,44,110,116,144
Tocopherol	134,246
Tolazamide	35,43,48,54,68,81,118,133,182,210, 218-224,264
Tolbutamide	35,43,48,54,68,81,118,133,182,210, 218-224,264
Tolmetin	13,18,80,85,131,139,144-147,148, 192,250
Torsemide	17,112,16-17,225,227
Tradalafil	29,78,109
Trandolapril	47,79-81,120,144,138,141,215, 218,247
TRANSPLANT IMMUNOSUPPRESSANTS	247-255
Tranylcypromine	77,115,153,157,175,180-182,184, 190,212,216,219,268
Triamcinolone	23,27,34,52,161,166,194,209, 242-245,258,259
Triazolam	26,30,56,66,92,148,,198-200,261
Trichlormethiazide	114,118,179,193,217,220
Tricyclic Antidepressants [Amitriptyline, Amoxapine, Clomipramine, Desipramine, Doxepin, Imipramine, Nortriptyline, Protriptyline, Trimipramine]	38,55,76,115,159,175,182,185,187, 189-191,243
Triethiodide	49
Trimethoprim	47,48,133,140,172,220,252
Trimethoprim/ Sulfamethoxazole	47-48

Trimipramine	38,55,76,115,159,175,182,185,187, 189-191,243
Troleandomycin	23-33,91,112,130,150,157,199,200, 229,243,250,255,256
Tromethamine	40,179,193,222
Trovafloxacin	25,33-38,60,90,100,101,104,107, 123,132,150,221,241,251
Tryptophan	269
Tubocurarine	49,97
Urecosuric Agents (Probenecid, Sulfinpyrazone)	12,15,22,44,65,139,146,210
Urinary Alkalinizers [Potassium Citrate, Sodium Acetate, Sodium Bicarbonate, Sodium Citrate, Sodium Lactate, Tromethamine]	40,179,193,222
Vaedenafil	29,78,109
Valproate Sodium	55,159,161,163,164,172,173-175, 190,210,225
Valproic Acid [Divalproex Sodium, Valproic Acid, Valproate Sodium]	55,159,161,163,164,172,173-175, 190,210,225
Valsartan	81,177,191
Vancomycin	49
Vardenafil	29,78,109
Vecuronium	49,97
Venlafaxine	145,159,178,182,183-192,213,234, 251,257,268,269
Verapamil	23,27,31,51,69,71,72,90-98,111, 115,165,171,232,236,237,248,250, 252
Vinca Alkaloids	26
Vincristine	26,110

Vitamin E (Tocopherol)	134,246
Vitamin K (Phytonadione) (Food Sourse)	247
Vitamin K Antagonists (Warfarin, Acenocoumarol)	14,20,22,30,33,35,36,43,47,55,68, 75, 100, 108,119,120,126-135, 142, 145, 152,160,164, 165, 197,208, 211, 222, 225,226, 223,231, 234,246,266,267
Voriconazole	66-74,90,107,164,197,198,200,228, 253,254,257
Warfarin	14,20,22,30,33,35,36,43,47,55,68, 75, 100, 108,119,120,126-135, 142, 145, 152,160,164, 165, 197,208, 211, 222, 225,226, 223,231, 234,246,266,267
Zidovudine	15,30,61,65
Zileuton	89,135,152
Zinc Gluconate	41
Zinc Salts	35
Zinc Sulfate	41
Zolmitriptan	269
Zolpidem	201

www.ingramcontent.com/pod-product-compliance
Lightning Source LLC
Chambersburg PA
CBHW031824170526
45157CB00001B/174